Frank Schneider (Hrsg./Ed.)

Psychiatrie im Nationalsozialismus

Erinnerung und Verantwortung

Psychiatry under National Socialism

Remembrance and Responsibility

Frank Schneider (Hrsg./Ed.)

Psychiatrie im Nationalsozialismus

Erinnerung und Verantwortung

Psychiatry under National Socialism

Remembrance and Responsibility

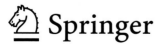 Springer

**Deutsche Gesellschaft für Psychiatrie,
Psychotherapie und Nervenheilkunde (DGPPN)**
Reinhardtstraße 4
D-10117 Berlin
www.dgppn.de

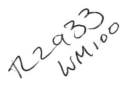

ISBN 978-3-642-20468-5   Springer-Verlag Berlin Heidelberg New York

Bibliografische Information der Deutschen Nationalbibliothek
Die Deutsche Nationalbibliothek verzeichnet diese Publikation in der Deutschen Nationalbibliografie;
detaillierte bibliografische Daten sind im Internet über http://dnb.d-nb.de abrufbar.

Springer Medizin
Springer-Verlag GmbH
Ein Unternehmen von Springer Science+Business Media
springer.de
© Deutsche Gesellschaft für Psychiatrie, Psychotherapie und Nervenheilkunde (DGPPN) Berlin 2011

Planung: Renate Scheddin, Heidelberg
Projektmanagement: Diana Kraplow, Heidelberg
Copy-Editing: Silvia Göhring, Iggelbach
Einbandgestaltung: deblik, Berlin
Satz: TypoStudio Tobias Schaedla, Heidelberg

SPIN 80053101
Gedruckt auf säurefreiem Papier   5141/DK – 5 4 3 2 1 0

Preface

On 14th July 1933 the National Socialists passed a "Law for the Prevention of Hereditarily Diseased Offspring", under which over 360 000 people, many of them mentally ill, were forcibly sterilised. Six years later, Hitler issued a decree (dated 1st September 1939) to launch a euphemistically dubbed "euthanasia" programme that later became known as "Aktion T4". This claimed the lives of 250 000 to 300 000 psychiatric patients and mentally and physically disabled people. German psychiatrists were instrumental in this programme and in many other atrocities committed during the Nazi era. Children were killed, ill people were deliberately starved, and experiments were performed on psychiatric patients before they were murdered and their brains dissected. Psychiatry under National Socialism was truly one of the darkest chapters in the history of the field.

It was only in the 1980s, after far too many years of silence, trivialisation, denial and continued discrimination against the victims and their families, that German psychiatry gradually began the painful and difficult process of coming to terms with this chapter of its past. Finally, almost 70 years after the atrocities committed by its members and officials, including its presidents, the German Association for Psychiatry and Psychotherapy (DGPPN) established a commission to address the actions of its predecessor associations during the "Third Reich" and, in 2009, amended its Articles of Association so that the first paragraph now explicitly acknowledges that the DGPPN has a special responsibility as a result of its predecessors' involvement in the crimes of National Socialism.

The annual convention of the DGPPN in Berlin in 2010 was dedicated to the victims of these crimes and to the issue of the association's responsibility. Around 3 000 psychiatrists gathered at the main commemorative event on 26th November 2010 to honour the memory of victims who were killed and subjected to ethically unjustifiable research and forced sterilisation, and of their colleagues who were forced into emigration. The speech held by the President of the DGPPN at the event is given here, as are the moving testimonies of the son of a Jewish psychiatrist forced into emigration and the niece of a woman who was forcibly sterilised and later killed. The enclosed DVD contains a recording of the event in the original German and a dubbed English version and includes a reading of historical documents and letters.

In light of the significance of this issue for the past, present and future of psychiatry, we decided to make these texts available in a dual-language book so they would be accessible to a broader international public. May this book serve as a constant reminder of the responsibility we psychiatrists have to the people entrusted to our care, and of our obligation to put individuals and their interests first, and, in all our words and deeds, never to forget the principles of humanity and the inviolability of human dignity.

Frank Schneider   *Aachen, summer 2011*

Vorwort

Am 14. Juli 1933 erließen die Nationalsozialisten das „Gesetz zur Verhütung erbkranken Nachwuchses". Es war die Grundlage für die zwangsweise Sterilisierung von über 360 000 kranken Menschen, darunter viele psychisch Erkrankte. Sechs Jahre später, datiert auf den 1. September 1939, befahl Hitler die von den Nazis euphemistisch so genannte „Euthanasie"-Aktion, später „T4"-Aktion, der 250 000 bis 300 000 psychisch, geistig und körperlich kranke Menschen zum Opfer fielen. An diesen Aktionen und vielen anderen schrecklichen Taten waren deutsche Psychiater maßgeblich beteiligt. Kinder wurden getötet, Kranke ließ man absichtlich verhungern, an psychiatrischen Patienten wurden Versuche durchgeführt, bevor sie ermordet und ihre Gehirne untersucht wurden. Die Psychiatrie im Nationalsozialismus zählt zu den dunkelsten Kapiteln der Geschichte des Fachgebietes.

Nach viel zu langen Jahren des Schweigens, des Kleinredens und Verdrängens und der fortdauernden Diskriminierung der Opfer und ihrer Angehörigen begann erst allmählich und unter großen Schwierigkeiten in den 1980er Jahren die Aufarbeitung dieser Zeit. Und fast 70 Jahre nach den Gräueltaten, die von ihren Mitgliedern und Funktionären, bis hin zu ihren Präsidenten, begangen wurden, hat die Deutsche Gesellschaft für Psychiatrie, Psychotherapie und Nervenheilkunde (DGPPN) eine Kommission zur Aufarbeitung ihrer Geschichte eingesetzt und ihrer Satzung im Jahr 2009 einen ersten Paragraphen vorangestellt, der ihre aus der Vergangenheit erwachsene Verantwortung konkret benennt.

Der Jahreskongress 2010 der DGPPN in Berlin war der Erinnerung an die Opfer und dieser Verantwortung der psychiatrischen Fachgesellschaft gewidmet. In der zentralen Gedenkveranstaltung am 26. November 2010 gedachten etwa 3 000 Psychiaterinnen und Psychiater der Opfer erzwungener Emigration, nicht zu rechtfertigender Forschung, der Zwangssterilisierung und der Ermordung psychisch erkrankter Menschen. Die Erklärung des Präsidenten der DGPPN wird hier dargestellt. Als Vertreter der Opfergruppen sprachen der Sohn eines emigrierten jüdischen Psychiaters und die Nichte einer zwangssterilisierten und schließlich ermordeten Patientin. Diese beeindruckenden Zeugnisse sind hier ebenfalls abgedruckt. Schließlich zeigt die beigefügte DVD in deutscher und synchronisierter englischer Fassung den gesamten Mitschnitt der Gedenkveranstaltung, einschließlich der Lesung aus historischen Briefen und Dokumenten.

Wir haben die Verbreitung dieser Texte in einer zweisprachigen Buchform gewählt, um sie angesichts der Bedeutung des Themas für Geschichte, Gegenwart und Zukunft der Psychiatrie einem möglichst breiten Publikum international zugänglich zu machen. Möge dieses Buch dazu beitragen, dass wir Psychiaterinnen und Psychiater uns unserer Verantwortung und einer humanen, am einzelnen Menschen orientierten Psychiatrie immer bewusst bleiben und sie in unserem Reden und in unserem Handeln nie vergessen.

Frank Schneider   *Aachen, im Sommer 2011*

❯ Speech of the President of the German Association for Psychiatry and Psychotherapy (DGPPN) Prof. Dr. Dr. Frank Schneider, Aachen

Ladies and Gentlemen!

Under National Socialism, psychiatrists showed contempt towards the patients in their care; they lied to them, and deceived them and their families. They forced them to be sterilised, arranged their deaths and even performed killings themselves. Patients were used as test subjects for unjustifiable research – research that left them traumatized or even dead.

Why has it taken us so long to face up to these facts and deal openly with this dark chapter in our history? Although we are proud that the German Association for Psychiatry and Psychotherapy (DGPPN) is one of the oldest scientific medical associations in the world, for too long now we have been hiding, denying a crucial part of our past. For that, we are truly ashamed.

It is also a disgrace that we, the DGPPN, did not even stand up for the victims in the period after 1945. Worse still, we were partially responsible for the renewed discrimination that they faced in the post-war period. We are at a loss to explain why we are only now in a position to hold an event such as this.

I stand before you today as President of an association that has taken nearly 70 years to end this silence and recall the tradition of enlightenment through science in which it stands. An independent scientific commission is currently overseeing a research project that is addressing the history of the association, or rather its predecessors, in the period between 1933 and 1945.

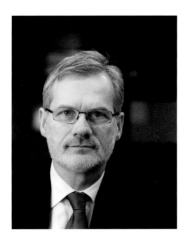

❯ Erklärung des Präsidenten der Deutschen Gesellschaft für Psychiatrie, Psychotherapie und Nervenheilkunde (DGPPN) Prof. Dr. Dr. Frank Schneider, Aachen

Sehr geehrte Damen und Herren,

Psychiater haben in der Zeit des Nationalsozialismus Menschen verachtet, die ihnen anvertrauten Patientinnen und Patienten in ihrem Vertrauen getäuscht und belogen, die Angehörigen hingehalten, Patienten zwangssterilisieren und töten lassen und auch selbst getötet. An Patienten wurde nicht zu rechtfertigende Forschung betrieben, Forschung, die Patienten schädigte oder gar tötete.

Warum haben wir so lange gebraucht, uns diesen Tatsachen zu stellen und offen mit diesem Teil unserer Geschichte umzugehen? Einerseits sind wir stolz, dass die DGPPN zu den ältesten wissenschaftlichen medizinischen Fachgesellschaften der Welt zählt. Andererseits wurde viel zu lange ein wichtiger Teil der Geschichte dieser Fachgesellschaft ausgeblendet, verdrängt. Dafür schämen wir uns.

Wir sind auch beschämt, weil wir, die deutsche psychiatrische Fachgesellschaft, nicht einmal in der Zeit nach 1945, an der Seite der Opfer gestanden haben. Schlimmer noch: Wir hatten Anteil an ihrer erneuten Diskriminierung und Benachteiligung. Uns fehlen noch die Worte, warum eine Veranstaltung wie diese erst heute möglich sein konnte.

Es hat fast 70 Jahre gedauert, bis sich die Fachgesellschaft, als deren Präsident ich heute hier vor Ihnen stehe, entschlossen hat, dieser Sprachlosigkeit ein Ende zu setzen und sich an ihre Tradition einer Aufklärung durch Wissenschaft zu erinnern. Eine wissenschaftliche Kommission, selbständig und unabhängig, begleitet derzeit ein Forschungsprojekt, um die Geschichte der Fachgesellschaft bzw. deren Vorläuferorganisationen zunächst in der Zeit zwischen 1933 und 1945 aufzuarbeiten.

But this is not enough. Irrespective of any research results, which we expect to receive in the next few years, I must offer our sincerest apologies – albeit shamefully late – to all the victims and their families who suffered such injustice and pain at the hands of the German associations and their psychiatrists.

The German Association for Psychiatry and Psychotherapy has decided to give a clear signal by holding this commemorative event as a way of acknowledging and of standing up for the victims, of coming to terms with our past and of learning from this bleak period in our history.

Ladies and gentlemen, welcome to this commemorative event. It is wonderful to see so many of you here and I would like to take this opportunity to thank you all for coming.

The letters and documents we have just heard at the beginning of this commemorative event provide moving testimonials of the pain and suffering that mentally ill people were subjected to.

Psychiatry under National Socialism is one of the darkest chapters in the history of our discipline. Throughout this period, psychiatrists and representatives of psychiatric associations repeatedly disregarded and heinously reinterpreted their professional duty to treat and care for their patients.

Aber das ist nicht genug: Unabhängig von den Forschungsergebnissen, die wir in den nächsten Jahren erwarten, habe ich – spät genug – bei allen Opfern und Angehörigen um Entschuldigung zu bitten für das erlittene Unrecht und Leid, das ihnen von deutschen Verbänden und ihren Psychiatern zugefügt wurde.

Die Deutsche Gesellschaft für Psychiatrie, Psychotherapie und Nervenheilkunde hat sich zu dieser Gedenkveranstaltung entschlossen, um ein deutliches Zeichen zu setzen, getragen von dem Willen, die Opfer anzuerkennen und an ihrer Seite zu stehen, sich zu der eigenen Vergangenheit zu bekennen und aus der Vergangenheit zu lernen.

Sehr geehrte Damen und Herren, ich begrüße Sie sehr herzlich zu dieser Gedenkveranstaltung und danke Ihnen, dass Sie so zahlreich gekommen sind.

Die Briefe und Dokumente, die wir eben gehört haben, geben ein eindrückliches Zeugnis von dem, was psychisch kranke Menschen erlitten haben und was ihnen angetan wurde.

Die Psychiatrie im Nationalsozialismus zählt zu den dunkelsten Kapiteln der Geschichte unseres Fachgebietes. Psychiater und die Vertreter ihrer Verbände haben in dieser Zeit ihren ärztlichen Auftrag, die ihnen anvertrauten Menschen zu heilen und zu pflegen, vielfach missachtet und eigenständig umgedeutet.

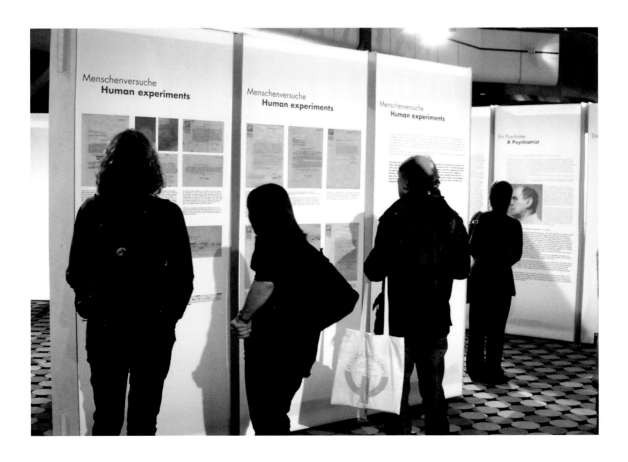

Psychiatry was corruptible and it corrupted, it cured and it killed. It no longer felt it had an obligation to individuals; rather, in the name of supposed progress – the liberation of an entire society from the burden of providing welfare, improvements in the genetic makeup of an entire nation and, ultimately, humanity's "deliverance from misery"[1] – psychiatrists abused and killed vast numbers of people. They also saw to it that any undesirable colleagues were forced out of their jobs.

It is important to remember that between 1933 and 1945 many of the psychiatrists working in academia emigrated from the Reich.[2] They did not leave voluntarily. Psychiatrists of Jewish descent or those who had the wrong political views were forced out of their jobs and had to stop practicing. They and their families lost their livelihoods, their belongings – and all too often their home country. Driven out of Germany, they had to create new lives for themselves as strangers in an unfamiliar, foreign land.

Most of those who could not flee Germany or Austria were deported to concentration or extermination camps. Few survived, and nothing we do can ever make up for the fate they suffered.

This was all happening at a time when psychiatric research in the Reich was becoming increasingly focused on eugenics and "racial hygiene".[3] National Socialist healthcare, social and economic policies favoured those who would most benefit the nation's health and productivity. The weak were to be eliminated so that the strong could become even stronger. This devastating approach was nothing new.

The term "eugenics" had been in use since the late 19th century[4], and the practice of sterilising mentally ill patients was being promoted in the Scandinavian and Anglo-Saxon countries as well as in the German Empire. In the summer of 1914 a proposed Bill on Sterilisation and Abortion was put forward in the Reichstag. It was only the outbreak of war that stopped the bill passing into law.[5]

---

[1] Title of a book by E. Mann published in 1922 by Fritz Fink Verlag, Weimar.

[2] Outlined in Zalashik R, Davidovitch N (2009) Professional identity across the borders: Refugee psychiatrists in Palestine, 1933–1945. Social History of Medicine 22: 569–587; Weindling P (2010) Alien Psychiatrists: The British assimilation of psychiatric refugees. In: Roelcke V, Weindling P, Westwood L (eds) International Relations in Psychiatry: Britain, America, and Germany to World War II. University of Rochester Press, Rochester/NY, pp 218–235.

[3] Roelcke V, Hohendorf G, Rotzoll M (2000) Psychiatric science, 'Euthanasia' and the 'new man': The debate on anthropological premises and values in national socialist medicine" ["Psychiatrische Wissenschaft, 'Euthanasie' und der 'Neue Mensch': Zur Diskussion um anthropologische Prämissen und Wertsetzungen in der Medizin im Nationalsozialismus]. In: Frewer A, Eickhoff C (eds) "Euthansia" and the current debate on assisted suicide. The historical background of medical ethics ["Euthanasie" und die aktuelle Sterbehilfe-Debatte. Die historischen Hintergründe medizinischer Ethik], Campus, Frankfurt/M., pp 193–217.

[4] Weingart P, Kroll J, Bayertz K (1988) Race, blood and genes [Rasse, Blut und Gene], Suhrkamp, Frankfurt/M., p 284; Nowak K (1980) Euthanasia" and sterilisations in the "Third Reich" ["Euthanasie" und Sterilisierungen im "Dritten Reich"]. Vandenhoeck & Ruprecht, Göttingen, p 39.

[5] Ganssmüller C (1987) The Third Reich's sterilisation law policy [Die Erbgesundheitspolitik des Dritten Reiches]. Böhlau, Cologne, p 13f.

Die Psychiatrie war verführbar und hat verführt, hat geheilt und vernichtet. Sie hat sich nicht mehr dem einzelnen Menschen verpflichtet gefühlt, sondern hat im Namen eines angeblichen Fortschritts, den man in der Befreiung einer ganzen Gesellschaft von Fürsorgelasten sah, in der Verbesserung der Erbanlagen eines Volkes und schließlich in der „Erlösung der Menschheit vom Elend"[1], massenhaft Menschen misshandelt und getötet – und unliebsame Kolleginnen und Kollegen aus ihren Ämtern gedrängt.

Wir haben uns zu vergegenwärtigen, dass in den Jahren von 1933 bis 1945 viele der akademisch tätigen Nervenärzte aus dem damaligen Deutschen Reich emigrierten.[2] Ihre Emigration erfolgte nicht freiwillig. Kolleginnen und Kollegen jüdischer Herkunft oder wegen ihrer politischen Überzeugung unliebsam gewordene Ärzte wurden aus ihren Ämtern und Funktionen gedrängt. Sie und ihre Angehörigen verloren ihre Anstellung und ihre Lebensgrundlage, ihr Hab und Gut – und nur zu oft auch ihre Heimat. Diese emigrierten Kolleginnen und Kollegen mussten sich mitsamt ihren Familien als Fremde in einem ihnen dann fremden Land eine neue Existenz aufbauen.

Die meisten derjenigen, die Deutschland oder Österreich nicht verlassen konnten, wurden im Krieg in die Konzentrations- und Vernichtungslager deportiert, ein Schicksal, das nur wenige überlebten. Dies ist nicht wieder gutzumachen.

Das alles geschah, während sich die psychiatrische Forschung im Deutschen Reich mehr und mehr auf eugenische und rassehygienische Themen konzentrierte.[3] Die Gesundheits-, Sozial- und Wirtschaftspolitik der nationalsozialistischen Weltanschauung zielte auf die Förderung derjenigen, die zur Gesundheit und Leistungsfähigkeit des Volkes beitragen konnten. Das Schwache sollte ausgeschieden werden, damit das Starke umso stärker wird. Dieses Denken steht in einer fatalen Tradition.

Schon seit dem ausgehenden 19. Jahrhundert wurde der Begriff Eugenik verwendet und die Sterilisation psychisch Kranker propagiert[4], im Deutschen Reich ebenso wie in Skandinavien und den angelsächsischen Ländern. Bereits im Sommer 1914 wurde ein Gesetzentwurf „für die Unfruchtbarmachung und Schwangerschaftsunterbrechung" in den deutschen Reichstag eingebracht. Nur der beginnende erste Weltkrieg verhinderte die weitere Beratung und Verabschiedung.[5]

---

[1] Titel des 1922 bei Fritz Fink, Weimar, erschienen Buches von E. Mann.

[2] Dargestellt in: Zalashik R, Davidovitch N (2009) Professional identity across the borders: Refugee psychiatrists in Palestine, 1933–1945. Social History of Medicine 22: 569–587; Weindling P (2010) Alien Psychiatrists: The British assimilation of psychiatric refugees. In: Roelcke V, Weindling P, Westwood L (Hrsg) International Relations in Psychiatry: Britain, America, and Germany to World War II. University of Rochester Press, Rochester/NY, S 218–235.

[3] Roelcke V, Hohendorf G, Rotzoll M (2000) Psychiatrische Wissenschaft, „Euthanasie" und der „Neue Mensch": Zur Diskussion um anthropologische Prämissen und Wertsetzungen in der Medizin im Nationalsozialismus. In: Frewer A, Eickhoff C (Hrsg) „Euthanasie" und die aktuelle Sterbehilfe-Debatte. Die historischen Hintergründe medizinischer Ethik. Campus, Frankfurt/M., S 193–217.

[4] Weingart P, Kroll J, Bayertz K (1988) Rasse, Blut und Gene. Suhrkamp, Frankfurt/M., S 284; Nowak K (1980) „Euthanasie" und Sterilisierung im „Dritten Reich". Vandenhoeck & Ruprecht, Göttingen, S 39.

[5] Ganssmüller C (1987) Die Erbgesundheitspolitik des Dritten Reiches. Böhlau, Köln, S 13f.

On 14th July 1933, not long after Hitler seized power, the NSDAP passed a Law for the Prevention of Hereditarily Diseased Offspring. The psychiatrist Ernst Rüdin, who was President of the psychiatric association from 1935 to 1945, was involved in writing the official commentary[6] to the law when he was director of the German Research Institute for Psychiatry.[7] The law described sterilisation – forced sterilisation – as "protecting future generations".[8] This is a truly perverse view that offsets one person's pain and suffering against another's wellbeing.

The law classed manic-depressive illness and schizophrenia as genetic mental illnesses. The same applied to many other conditions, such as hereditary forms of epilepsy, blindness, deafness, dwarfism, etc. The idea was to stop sick people having children so that their supposedly bad genetic material did not continue to pollute the health of the "Volk".

---

[6] Gütt A, Rüdin R, Ruttke F (1936) Law for the prevention of heriditarily diseased offspring of 14 June 1933, with implementing ordinances [Gesetz zur Verhütung erbkranken Nachwuchses vom 14. Juni 1933 nebst Ausführungsverordnungen]. J.F. Lehmanns, Munich, 2nd edition.

[7] Roelcke V (2008) Science in the service of the Reich: Ernst Rüdin and the German Institute for Psychiatric Research [Wissenschaft im Dienst des Reiches: Ernst Rüdin und die Deutsche Forschungsanstalt für Psychiatrie]. In: Hockerts G, Hajak S (eds) Munich and national socialism [München und der Nationalsozialismus]. Metropol, Berlin, pp 313–331.

[8] loc. cit., p 5, in the preface to the first edition of 1934 (note 6).

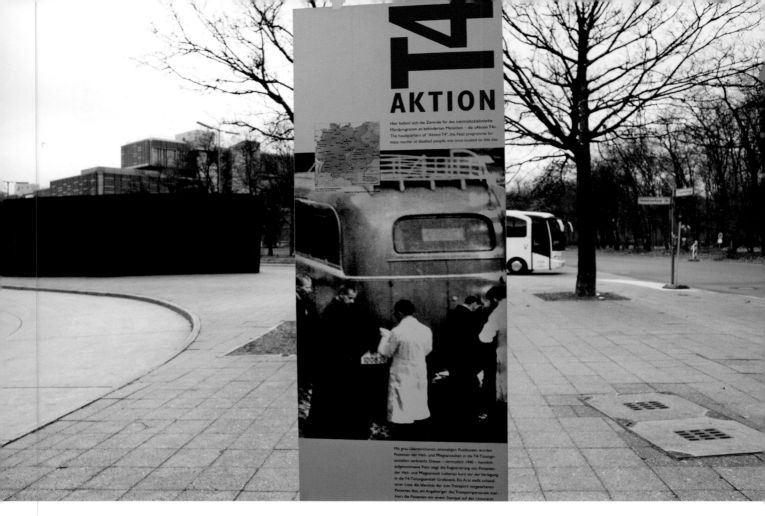

Berlin, Tiergartenstraße 4

Am 14. Juli 1933, nur kurze Zeit nach der von der NSDAP selbst so genannten „Machtergreifung" Hitlers, wurde dann das „Gesetz zur Verhütung erbkranken Nachwuchses" verabschiedet, an dessen offiziellem Kommentar[6] der Psychiater – und in den Jahren 1935–1945 Präsident der psychiatrischen Gesellschaft – Ernst Rüdin, damals Direktor der Deutschen Forschungsanstalt für Psychiatrie, mitgewirkt hat.[7] Die Sterilisierung, die zwangsweise Sterilisierung, wurde darin als „Vorsorge für das kommende Geschlecht"[8] bezeichnet. Eine perverse Darstellung, denn sie rechnet Leid und Verletzung der einen gegen das Wohl der anderen auf.

Im Gesetz wurden manisch-depressive Erkrankungen und Schizophrenie als solche vererbbaren psychischen Erkrankungen genannt, ebenso aber auch erbliche Formen der Epilepsie sowie der Blind- und Taubheit, Kleinwuchs und vieles mehr. Kranke Menschen sollten keine Kinder zeugen. Ihr für schlecht befundenes Genmaterial sollte so den gesunden „Volkskörper" nicht weiter belasten.

---

[6] Gütt A, Rüdin R, Ruttke F (1936) Gesetz zur Verhütung erbkranken Nachwuchses vom 14. Juni 1933 nebst Ausführungsverordnungen. J.F. Lehmanns, München, 2. Auflage.

[7] Roelcke V (2008) Wissenschaft im Dienst des Reiches: Ernst Rüdin und die Deutsche Forschungsanstalt für Psychiatrie. In: Hockerts G, Hajak S (Hrsg) München und der Nationalsozialismus. Metropol, Berlin, S 313–331.

[8] a.a.O., S 5, im Vorwort zur 1. Auflage von 1934 (s. Fußnote 6).

All doctors were obliged to report "hereditarily diseased" individuals to the authorities. Under the law, doctors forcibly sterilised more than 360 000 people. Over 6 000 died as a consequence of the operations.

Since the concepts of eugenics and racial hygiene were so popular at the time, many psychiatrists held the sterilisation law in high regard. As President of our predecessor organisation, the Society of German Neurologists and Psychiatrists (GDNP), Ernst Rüdin spoke in its favour several times at the openings of annual congresses.[9] Other countries around the world also supported eugenics-based sterilisation. However, what set Germany apart was the fact that its law allowed people to be sterilised against their will. For its victims, the legislation was an appalling attack on the very core of their identity – an attack they were powerless to stop and that permanently robbed them of their right to physical integrity and to parenthood.

Even once the war had ended, shame and silence continued to shroud what the victims and their families had endured. To this day the Federal Republic of Germany has still not formally recognised these individuals as victims of Nazi persecution, despite the fact that the sterilisation law was an unequivocal expression of National Socialist, German racial ideology. The commentary to the law makes this very clear:

"What is the aim of measures for the genetic and racial hygiene adequate for the German Volk? The existence at all times of a sufficient number of genetically healthy large families that are racially valuable to the German people."[10]

At this point I would like to express my admiration for Dorothea Buck. The sculptor and author, who was herself one of the victims, co-founded the "Federal Organisation of (Ex-)Users of Psychiatry" in Germany. She has tirelessly dedicated herself to raising awareness of the issues and to ensuring that they are not forgotten. Klara Nowak, who passed away years ago, was another such person. Ms Nowak's 1987 initiative resulted in the creation of the "Federation of Those Affected by 'Euthanasia' and Forced Sterilisation" which since then fought for the social rehabilitation of victims.

Yet the violence did not end at forced sterilisation – people were also murdered. In the 1920s, as a result of the World War and the Great Depression, disabled people began to be seen as financial burdens. Psychiatrist Alfred Erich Hoche published *Allowing the Destruction of Life Unworthy of Living* in 1920 in collaboration with the lawyer Karl Binding. In it, he coined the term "human ballast" and drew up a list of allegedly incurable mental illnesses that rendered

---

[9] Rüdin E (1939) The importance of research and cooperation of neurologists and psychiatrists in the national socialist state [Bedeutung der Forschung und Mitarbeit von Neurologen und Psychiatern im nationalsozialistischen Staat]. Zeitschrift für die gesamte Neurologie und Psychiatrie 165: 7–17.

[10] It continues: "However, this goal can only be achieved and ensured over the long term if the concept of breeding remains at the core of our concept of racial hygiene. The future keepers of the law must bear in mind the aim of ensuring the bloodstock of the German people […] remains pure." loc. cit., p 55 (note 6).

Alle Ärzte wurden verpflichtet, diese sog. „Erbkranken" gegenüber den Behörden anzuzeigen. Über 360 000 Menschen wurden auf Grundlage dieses Gesetzes von Medizinern selektiert und zwangssterilisiert. Über 6 000 starben bei den Eingriffen.

Vor dem Hintergrund eugenischer und rassehygienischer Denkweisen galten die Sterilisationsgesetze bei vielen Psychiatern als vorbildlich. Ernst Rüdin hat sich als Präsident unserer Vorläuferorganisation mehrfach bei der Eröffnung der Jahrestagungen der GDPN dafür ausgesprochen.[9] Und auch in anderen Ländern weltweit wurden Sterilisierungen auf eugenischer Grundlage befürwortet. In Deutschland erlaubte das Gesetz allerdings die Sterilisation auch gegen den Willen der Betroffenen. Für die Opfer war sie ein massiver, ein schrecklicher Eingriff in den Kernbereich ihrer Identität, dem sie ohnmächtig ausgeliefert waren. Sie wurden damit nicht nur unwiederbringlich ihres Rechts auf körperliche Unversehrtheit beraubt, sondern auch ihres Rechts auf Elternschaft.

Auch nach dem Krieg blieben den Opfern und ihren Familien in der Regel nur Scham und Schweigen über das, was ihnen angetan wurde. Und bis heute sind sie von der Bundesrepublik Deutschland nicht ausdrücklich als Opfer nationalsozialistischer Verfolgung anerkannt, obwohl doch das Sterilisationsgesetz explizit Ausdruck nationalsozialistischer, deutscher Rasseideologie war, wie im Kommentar zum Gesetz sehr deutlich wird. Dort heißt es:

„Welches ist nun das Ziel der dem deutschen Volk artgemäßen Erb- und Rassenpflege: Eine ausreichende Zahl Erbgesunder, für das deutsche Volk rassisch wertvoller, kinderreicher Familien zu allen Zeiten."[10]

Mit Bewunderung anerkennen möchte ich hier das spätere Engagement von Frau Dorothea Buck, Bildhauerin und Autorin, selbst Betroffene und Mitgründerin des Bundesverbands Psychiatrie-Erfahrener. Sie hat immer wieder aufgeklärt, gemahnt und erinnert, ebenso wie Klara Nowak, die vor Jahren verstarb. Frau Nowaks Initiative ist es zu verdanken, dass sich 1987 Zwangssterilisierte und „Euthanasie"-Geschädigte zusammenfanden und den Bund der „Euthanasie"-Geschädigten und Zwangssterilisierten gründeten, der seitdem um die gesellschaftliche Rehabilitation der Opfer gekämpft hat.

Aber es wurde nicht nur zwangssterilisiert, es wurde auch getötet. Schon in den 1920er Jahren wurden unter dem Eindruck des ersten Weltkriegs und der Weltwirtschaftskrise Kranke zu Kostenfaktoren. Es war ein Psychiater, Alfred Erich Hoche, der in seinem 1920 erschienenen Buch zur Freigabe der Vernichtung „lebensunwerten Lebens" gemeinsam mit dem Juristen Karl Binding den Begriff „Ballastexistenzen" prägte und einen Katalog angeblich unheilbarer psychi-

---

9 Rüdin E (1939) Bedeutung der Forschung und Mitarbeit von Neurologen und Psychiatern im nationalsozialistischen Staat. Zeitschrift für die gesamte Neurologie und Psychiatrie 165: 7–17.

10 Und weiter: „Dieses Ziel ist jedoch nur dann zu erreichen und für die Dauer sicherzustellen, wenn der Zuchtgedanke Kerngehalt des Rassegedankens bleibt. Die künftigen Rechtswahrer müssen sich über das Zuchtziel des deutschen Volkes […] klar sein." a.a.O., S 55 (s. Fußnote 6).

sufferers "mentally dead".[11] This provided the basis for the call for "death to life unworthy of life!" published in 1930 in the National Socialist monthly bulletin.[12]

Later, Hitler issued a decree to start a "euthanasia" programme. It was backdated to 1st September 1939, the date that Germany invaded Poland and World War II began. Professor Werner Heyde, chair of psychiatry and neurology of Würzburg University, was appointed Medical Director of the programme that would later become known as "Aktion T4". It is thought that, by the end of the war – and even several weeks afterwards – Aktion T4 and the killings that took place once the programme had officially ended claimed the lives of at least 250 000 to 300 000 mentally and physically disabled people.[13]

---

[11] Binding K, Hoche A (1920) Allowing the destruction of life unworthy of living. To what extent and in what form [Die Freigabe der Vernichtung lebensunwerten Lebens. Ihr Maß und ihre Form]. Meiner, Leipzig, 1920 (2nd edition 1922), p 57, cited in Nowak K, loc. cit., p 51 (note 4).

[12] Nationalsozialistische Monatshefte 1, 1930, p 298, cited in Nowak K, loc. cit. p 43.

[13] Faulstich H (2000) The number of 'Euthanasia' victims [Die Zahl der 'Euthanasie'-Opfer]. In: Frewer A, Eickhoff C (eds) „Euthanasia" and the current debate on assisted suicide. The historical background to medical ethics [Euthanasie und die aktuelle Sterbehilfe-Debatte. Die historischen Hintergründe medizinischer Ethik]. Campus, Frankfurt/M., pp 218–234.

scher Krankheiten erstellte, die er „Zustände geistigen Todes" nannte.[11] 1930 wurde daraus in den Nationalsozialistischen Monatsheften die Forderung: „Tod dem lebensunwerten Leben!"[12]

Rückdatiert auf den Überfall Deutschlands auf Polen, den Kriegsbeginn am 1. September 1939, befahl Hitler die sog. „Euthanasie"-Aktion. Zum medizinischen Leiter dieser später „Aktion T4" genannten Aktion wurde ein Psychiater und Neurologe, der Würzburger Ordinarius Professor Werner Heyde, bestimmt. Ihr und den nach ihrer offiziellen Beendigung sich anschließenden weiteren Phasen der Krankentötungen sollten bis zum Kriegsende – und noch einige Wochen darüber hinaus – mindestens 250 000 bis 300 000 psychisch, geistig und körperlich kranke Menschen zum Opfer fallen.[13]

---

[11] Binding K, Hoche A (1920) Die Freigabe der Vernichtung lebensunwerten Lebens. Ihr Maß und ihre Form. Meiner, Leipzig, 1920 (2. Auflage 1922), S 57, nach Nowak K, a.a.O. (s. Fußnote 4), S 51.

[12] Nationalsozialistische Monatshefte 1, 1930, S 298, nach Nowak K, a.a.O., S 43.

[13] Faulstich H (2000) Die Zahl der „Euthanasie"-Opfer. In: Frewer A, Eickhoff C (Hrsg) Euthanasie und die aktuelle Sterbehilfe-Debatte. Die historischen Hintergründe medizinischer Ethik. Campus, Frankfurt/M., S 218–234.

From October 1939, all psychiatric hospitals and associated areas in the Reich received registration forms from Columbushaus on Potsdamer Platz, and as of April 1940 from Tiergartenstraße 4, where the Berlin Philharmonic stands today. The forms were used to systematically record all patients and select who should die. Decisions were mainly based on "usefulness" criteria, that is, on how much work a person was capable of.[14]

Today, at the site of the former central administration-office for the killings all that commemorates the "euthanasia" victims is an indistinct plaque in the ground and a sculpture that was only dedicated to them upon completion. There is still no central, national memorial to the victims. This is a clear expression of the continuing denial surrounding the events, and of the humiliation that the survivors and their families still endure. It also represents a blind spot in the collective memory of our country and of German psychiatry. We at the DGPPN will be supporting current efforts to establish an appropriate national T4 commemorative and information centre.

Approximately fifty selected assessors, some of them renowned psychiatrists, evaluated the registration forms they received from the hospitals and decided who would live and who would die. Among the assessors were Werner Villinger, Friedrich Mauz and Friedrich Panse, all of whom held the office of President in our association during the post-war period.[15] Friedrich Mauz and Friedrich Panse also later became honorary members. Although membership ends with the death of the individual, we condemn both these cases and will formally revoke the honours.

Patients selected for death would be collected from their hospitals in grey buses that have now come to symbolise the killings, and taken to one of six mental institutions equipped with gas chambers. Medical facilities thus became extermination centres. Healing became destruction. Psychiatrists watched as the patients entrusted to their care were taken away to be murdered. In the order they were established, the six institutions were: Grafeneck, Brandenburg, Hartheim, Pirna-Sonnenstein, Bernburg, and Hadamar.

"Aktion T4" lasted nearly two years, from January 1940 to August 1941. Within that time, over 70 000 patients were killed. The public protests that eventually spelled the demise of the programme did not come from the ranks of the psychiatric profession, but predominantly from the Church. The crucial sermon against the killing-program was delivered on 3rd August 1941 by Clemens August Graf von Galen, Bishop of Munster and Cardinal of the Roman Catholic Church. "Aktion T4" was officially stopped immediately afterwards.[16]

---

[14] Rotzoll M, Hohendorf G, Fuchs P et al. (2010) The national socialist "Euthanasia" campaign "Aktion T4" and its victims [Die nationalsozialistische "Euthanasie"-Aktion "T4" und ihre Opfer]. Schöningh, Paderborn.

[15] Schmuhl H-W (1987) Racial hygiene, national socialism, euthanasia: From contraception to the destruction of "life unworthy of living" 1890–1945 [Rassenhygiene, Nationalsozialismus, Euthanasie: Von der Verhütung zur Vernichtung "lebensunwerten Lebens" 1890–1945]. Vandenhoeck & Ruprecht, Göttingen, p 192.

[16] Cf. Schmuhl, Racial hygiene [Rassenhygiene], pp 210–214.

Ab Oktober 1939 wurden zuerst aus dem Columbushaus am Potsdamer Platz, dann ab April 1940 aus der Tiergartenstraße 4, also dort, wo heute die Berliner Philharmonie steht, Meldebögen an die Heil- und Pflegeanstalten des Deutschen Reiches und der angegliederten Gebiete verschickt, um alle Patienten systematisch zu erfassen und zu selektieren. Die Selektion erfolgte wesentlich nach Nützlichkeitskriterien, also der Frage nach der Arbeitsleistung.[14]

Am Ort der ehemaligen Zentraldienststelle befinden sich heute nur eine unscheinbare, in den Boden eingelassene Gedenktafel für die „Euthanasie"-Opfer und eine erst nachträglich den Opfern gewidmete Plastik. Einen zentralen, nationalen Gedenkort für die Opfer der sog. „Euthanasie" gibt es weiterhin nicht. Das ist nicht nur für die Überlebenden und ihre Angehörigen Ausdruck fortdauernder Verdrängung und Erniedrigung, es ist auch ein blinder Fleck im Gedächtnis unseres Landes und der deutschen Psychiatrie. Die aktuelle Initiative zur Errichtung einer angemessenen nationalen „T4"-Gedenk- und Informationsstätte werden wir als Fachgesellschaft unterstützen.

Etwa 50 ausgewählte Gutachter, darunter damals namhafte Psychiater, werteten die von den Psychiatern der Kliniken zurückgeschickten Meldebögen aus, selektierten und entschieden über Leben und Tod. Unter diesen Gutachtern waren auch Werner Villinger, Friedrich Mauz und Friedrich Panse, in der Nachkriegszeit drei Präsidenten unserer Fachgesellschaft.[15] Friedrich Mauz und Friedrich Panse wurden später sogar Ehrenmitglieder unserer Gesellschaft. Zwar endet jede Ehrenmitgliedschaft der DGPPN mit dem Tod der Geehrten, wir verurteilen aber heute diese Ehrenmitgliedschaften und werden sie auch formal annullieren.

Mit grauen Bussen, dem bildhaften Symbol für das Töten, wurden die Patientinnen und Patienten aus den Heil- und Pflegeanstalten abgeholt und in sechs psychiatrische Anstalten gebracht, in denen Gaskammern eingerichtet worden waren. Heilanstalten wurden zu Vernichtungsanstalten. Aus Heilung wurde Vernichtung – und Psychiater überwachten den Abtransport und die Ermordung der ihnen anvertrauten Patienten. Die sechs Anstalten waren in der Reihenfolge ihrer Einrichtung: Grafeneck, Brandenburg, Hartheim, Pirna-Sonnenstein, Bernburg und Hadamar.

Innerhalb der knapp zwei Jahre, die die „T4"-Aktion offiziell andauerte, von Januar 1940 bis August 1941, wurden mehr als 70 000 Patienten ermordet. Und es waren nicht die Psychiater, die durch öffentlichen Protest zum Ende der „T4"-Aktion beitrugen. Der Protest kam vor allem aus den Kirchen. Die entscheidende Protestpredigt hielt Clemens August Kardinal von Galen, Bischof von Münster, am 3. August 1941. Unmittelbar danach wurde die „T4"-Aktion offiziell eingestellt.[16]

---

[14] Rotzoll M, Hohendorf G, Fuchs P et al. (Hrsg) (2010) Die nationalsozialistische „Euthanasie"-Aktion „T4" und ihre Opfer. Schöningh, Paderborn.

[15] Schmuhl H-W (1987) Rassenhygiene, Nationalsozialismus, Euthanasie: Von der Verhütung zur Vernichtung „lebensunwerten Lebens", 1890–1945. Vandenhoeck & Ruprecht, Göttingen, S 192.

[16] Vgl. Schmuhl, Rassenhygiene, S 210–214.

But the Nazis took the knowledge and experience gathered during "Aktion T4" and applied them to the concentration camps to murder even more people – this time in their millions.[17]

At the same time as they were implementing Aktion T4, the Nazis were also murdering physically and mentally disabled children in over 30 psychiatric and paediatric hospitals as part of what is usually called "child euthanasia". Previously it was thought that approximately 5 000 children had died. This figure was given by the perpetrators during post-war trials and then generally accepted as true. We now know that the actual number was far greater.

And yet the killing continued, even after the centrally organised "Aktion T4" was officially stopped. During this decentralised phase of "euthanasia", doctors in psychiatric facilities seeking to free up beds and save money killed patients – possibly many 10 000 – by administering overdoses or providing them with so little food that they starved to death.[18] In a report on new admissions in 1943, Gerhard Wischer, director of the Waldheim psychiatric hospital, put it very succinctly:

"Of course I could never accommodate the new patients without undertaking certain measures to free up space. The process itself is very straightforward, but there is a distinct shortage of the necessary medication."[19]

Today it is hard to imagine that psychiatrists allowed patients in their care to be killed, that they chose who should live or die and then medically, scientifically – well, pseudo-scientifically – oversaw the deaths of children, adults and elderly people.

An entry in a medical file from 1939 on a female patient suffering from a schizophrenic disorder, which is archived at the Federal Archives here in Berlin, reads as follows:

"As before. Mentally dead. No change can be expected, so medical record should be closed. The only entry worth making is the date of death".[20]

---

17 Friedlander H (1995) The origins of Nazi genocide: From euthanasia to the final solution. University of North Carolina Press, Chapel Hill.

18 Outlined in Faulstich H (1998) Starvation in psychiatry 1914–1949. With a topography of Nazi psychiatry [Hungersterben in der Psychiatrie 1914–1949. Mit einer Topographie der NS-Psychiatrie]. Lambertus, Freiburg/Br.; for a local example, cf. Schwarz P (2002) Murder by starvation, 'wild Euthanasia', and 'Aktion Brandt' at Steinhof during national socialism [Mord durch Hunger. Wilde 'Euthanasie' und 'Aktion Brandt' am Steinhof in der NS-Zeit]. In: Gabriel E, Neugebauer W (eds) From forced sterilisation to murder [Von der Zwangssterilisierung zur Ermordung]. Böhlau, Vienna, pp 113–142.

19 Letter of 4 Nov. 1943 from Dr. Wischer to Professor Nitsche, head of Central Department I, cited in Schmuhl, Racial hygiene [Rassenhygiene], 1992, p 232 (cf. Aly G (1985) Medicine against the useless [Medizin gegen Unbrauchbare]. Beiträge zur Nationalsozialistischen Gesundheits- und Sozialpolitik 1: 9–74, specifically p 61); cf. also Klee E (1983)" Euthanasia" in the Nazi state ["Euthanasie" im NS-Staat]. S. Fischer, Frankfurt/M., p 427.

20 Federal Archives Berlin R 179/24884, cited in Rotzoll M, Fuchs P, Richter P, Hohendorf G (2010) The national socialist 'Euthanasia' campaign 'Aktion T4' [Die nationalsozialistische 'Euthanasieaktion T4']. Nervenarzt 81: 1326–1332, specifically p 1331.

Das Wissen und die Erfahrungen, die im Zuge der „T4"-Aktion mit dem Töten gemacht wurden, nutzte man später in den Konzentrationslagern, um weitere Menschen, dieses Mal Millionen, zu ermorden.[17]

Parallel zur „Aktion T4" wurden im Zuge der sog. „Kinder-Euthanasie" in über 30 psychiatrischen und pädiatrischen Kliniken körperlich und psychisch kranke Kinder ermordet. Bisher ging man von ca. 5 000 Kindern aus, eine Zahl, die in den Nachkriegsprozessen von den Tätern selbst genannt und dann zunächst weitgehend unkritisch übernommen wurde. Wie sich jetzt herausstellt, ist sie viel zu gering angesetzt.

Aber es ist immer noch nicht genug, denn auch nach dem offiziellen Ende der zentral organisierten „T4"-Aktion ging das Töten weiter. In dieser dezentralen Phase der „Euthanasie" wurden in psychiatrischen Einrichtungen die Patienten – wahrscheinlich viele Zehntausende – durch eine Überdosis Medikamente getötet oder systematisch verhungert, um Bettenplätze zu schaffen und Geld einzusparen. Die Patienten erhielten Nahrung, aber nur gerade genug, um zu sterben.[18] Der Direktor der Heil- und Pflegeanstalt Waldheim, Gerhard Wischer, berichtet 1943 im Zusammenhang mit Neuaufnahmen ganz lapidar:

„Ich könnte diese Aufnahmen natürlich niemals unterbringen, wenn ich nicht entsprechende Maßnahmen zum Freimachen von Plätzen durchführen würde, was ganz reibungslos geht. Es fehlt mir allerdings sehr an den erforderlichen Medikamenten."[19]

All dies ist heute unvorstellbar, dass Psychiater ihre Patienten, die ihnen zur Heilung und Pflege anvertrauten Menschen, der Tötung preisgaben, dass sie sie selektierten und die Tötung selbst dann medizinisch, wissenschaftlich – pseudowissenschaftlich – überwachten: die Ermordung von Kindern, Erwachsenen und alten Menschen.

Ein ärztlicher Akteneintrag von 1939 über eine an einer schizophrenen Psychose erkrankte Patientin, der im Bundesarchiv hier in Berlin archiviert ist, lautet:

„Weiter so. Geistig tot. Das Krankenblatt sollte abgeschlossen werden, da sich auch in Zukunft nichts ändern wird. Der einzige Eintrag, der sich lohnt, ist die Notiz des Sterbedatums".[20]

---

[17] Friedlander H (1995) The origins of Nazi genocide: From euthanasia to the final solution. University of North Carolina Press, Chapel Hill.

[18] Dargestellt in Faulstich H (1998) Hungersterben in der Psychiatrie 1914–1949. Mit einer Topographie der NS-Psychiatrie. Lambertus, Freiburg/Br.; als lokales Beispiel, vgl. Schwarz P (2002) Mord durch Hunger, ‚Wilde Euthanasie' und ‚Aktion Brandt' am Steinhof in der NS-Zeit. In: Gabriel E, Neugebauer W (Hrsg) Von der Zwangssterilisierung zur Ermordung. Böhlau, Wien, S 113–142.

[19] Brief von Dr. Wischer an Professor Nitsche, Leiter der Hauptabteilung I, vom 4.11.1943, nach Schmuhl, Rassenhygiene, 1992, S 232 (vgl. Aly G (1985) Medizin gegen Unbrauchbare. Beiträge zur Nationalsozialistischen Gesundheits- und Sozialpolitik 1: 9–74, dort S 61, s. auch Klee E (1983) „Euthanasie" im NS-Staat. S. Fischer, Frankfurt/M., S 427.

[20] Bundesarchiv Berlin R 179/24884 nach Rotzoll M, Fuchs P, Richter P, Hohendorf G (2010) Die nationalsozialistische „Euthanasieaktion T4". Nervenarzt 81: 1326–1332, dort S 1331.

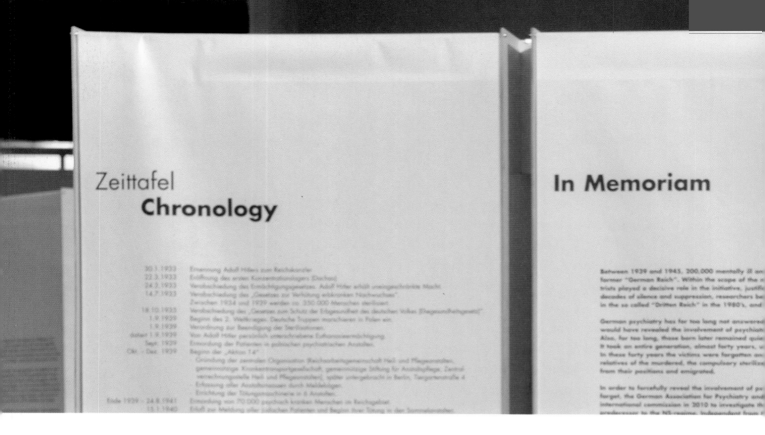

Before they were murdered, many patients were used for "research". This involved ethically unjustifiable experiments that are far removed from scientific and research values. One example is the "euthanasia"-related experiments on mentally ill children and teenagers by Carl Schneider, Chair and Professor of Psychiatry at Heidelberg University, in collaboration with Julius Deussen, an employee at the German Research Institute for Psychiatry in Munich. The research involved elaborate experiments on patients, followed by their killing and autopsies.[21] Patients at psychiatric hospitals were also used as test subjects in TB vaccination trials in Kaufbeuren[22], in work on the viral aetiology of multiple sclerosis in Werneck[23], and in neuropathological examinations on "euthanasia" victims who had probably been selected especially for this purpose. This was the project Julius Hallervorden carried out at the Kaiser Wilhelm Institute for Brain Research in Berlin-Buch in collaboration with the Brandenburg-Görden asylum, which was run by psychiatrist Hans Heinze.[24]

---

[21] Roelcke V (2000) Psychiatric science in the context of national socialist policy and 'Euthanasia': The role of Ernst Rüdin and the German Institute for Psychiatric Research [Psychiatrische Wissenschaft im Kontext nationalsozialistischer Politik und 'Euthanasie': Zur Rolle von Ernst Rüdin und der Deutschen Forschungsanstalt für Psychiatrie]. In: Kaufmann D (ed) The Kaiser Wilhelm Society under national socialism [Die Kaiser-Wilhelm-Gesellschaft im Nationalsozialismus]. Wallstein, Göttingen, pp 112–150; Roelcke V, Hohendorf G, Rotzoll M (1998) Research into hereditary psychology in the context of 'Euthanasia': New documents and perspectives on Carl Schneider, Julius Deussen and Ernst Rüdin [Erbpsychologische Forschung im Kontext der 'Euthanasie': Neue Dokumente und Aspekte zu Carl Schneider, Julius Deussen und Ernst Rüdin]. Fortschritte der Neurologie und Psychiatrie 66: 331–336.

[22] Dahl M (2002) "…whom keeping alive would not benefit the nation" ["deren Lebenserhaltung für die Nation keinen Vorteil bedeutet"]. In: Disabled children as test subjects and the development of the tuberculosis vaccination [Behinderte Kinder als Versuchsobjekte und die Entwicklung der Tuberkulose-Schutzimpfung]. Medizinhistorisches Journal 37: 57–90; cf. also von Cranach M, Siemen L (1999) Psychiatry under national socialism: Bavarian psychiatric hospitals and psychiatric asylums between 1933 and 1945 [Psychiatrie im Nationalsozialismus: Die Bayerischen Heil- und Pflegeanstalten zwischen 1933 und 1945]. Oldenbourg, Munich.

[23] Peiffer J (1998) Neurology in the 'Third Reich' [Neurologie im 'Dritten Reich']. Nervenarzt 69: 728–733.

[24] Shevell MI, Peiffer J (2001) Julius Hallervorden's wartime activities. Implications for science under dictatorship". Pediatric Neurology 25: 162–165.

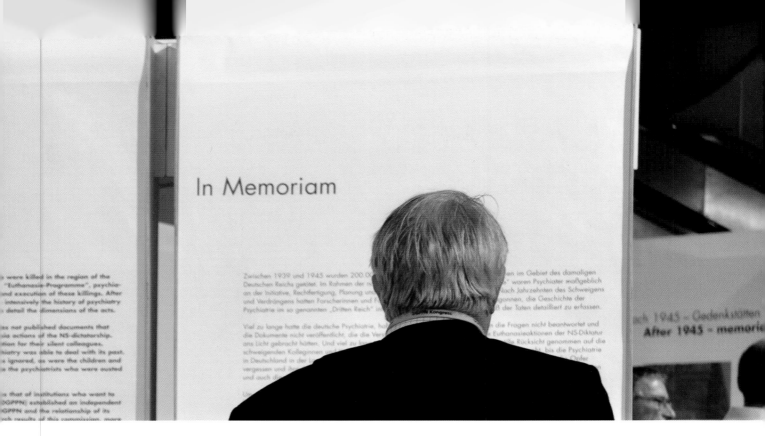

Vor der Ermordung wurde an vielen Patientinnen und Patienten „geforscht"; es handelte sich dabei um ethisch nicht zu rechtfertigende Experimente, die nichts mit den Werten von Wissenschaft und Forschung gemein haben. Beispiele sind die Arbeiten an psychisch kranken Kindern und Jugendlichen im Kontext der „Euthanasie" von Carl Schneider, Lehrstuhlinhaber für Psychiatrie in Heidelberg, in Kooperation mit Julius Deussen, einem Mitarbeiter der Deutschen Forschungsanstalt für Psychiatrie in München. Es handelte sich um aufwendige Experimente an Patienten und dann um ihre Tötung und Obduktion.[21] Auch wurden Untersuchungen an Patienten aus Heil- und Pflegeanstalten durchgeführt, z. B. TBC-Impfversuche in Kaufbeuren[22], Arbeiten zur Virusgenese der Multiplen Sklerose in Werneck[23] oder auch neuropathologische Untersuchungen an Euthanasie-Opfern, die wahrscheinlich speziell für diese Untersuchungen zur Euthanasie selektiert wurden. Dies geschah so durch Julius Hallervorden am Kaiser-Wilhelm-Institut für Hirnforschung in Kooperation mit der Anstalt Brandenburg-Görden unter der Leitung des Psychiaters Hans Heinze.[24]

[21] Roelcke V (2000) Psychiatrische Wissenschaft im Kontext nationalsozialistischer Politik und „Euthanasie": Zur Rolle von Ernst Rüdin und der Deutschen Forschungsanstalt für Psychiatrie. In: Kaufmann D (Hrsg) Die Kaiser-Wilhelm-Gesellschaft im Nationalsozialismus. Wallstein, Göttingen, S 112–150; Roelcke V, Hohendorf G, Rotzoll M (1998) Erbpsychologische Forschung im Kontext der „Euthanasie": Neue Dokumente und Aspekte zu Carl Schneider, Julius Deussen und Ernst Rüdin. Fortschritte der Neurologie und Psychiatrie 66: 331–336.

[22] Dahl M (2002) „…deren Lebenserhaltung für die Nation keinen Vorteil bedeutet": Behinderte Kinder als Versuchsobjekte und die Entwicklung der Tuberkulose-Schutzimpfung. Medizinhistorisches Journal 37: 57–90; s. auch von Cranach M, Siemen L (1999) Psychiatrie im Nationalsozialismus: Die Bayerischen Heil- und Pflegeanstalten zwischen 1933 und 1945. Oldenbourg, München.

[23] Peiffer J (1998) Neurologie im „Dritten Reich". Nervenarzt 69: 728–733.

[24] Shevell MI, Peiffer J (2001) Julius Hallervorden's wartime activities. Implications for science under dictatorship. Pediatric Neurology 25: 162–165.

The murdered patients' bodies and individual histopathological specimens were in high demand among scientists, and the research findings gained were being published even after the war ended. The Kaiser Wilhelm Institute for Brain Research used the brains of at least 295 "euthanasia" victims in its work[25], and even until recently there have been almost no qualms about using specimens taken from patients murdered during the Third Reich.[26]

The research was not confined to mental institutions. Tübingen-based psychiatrist Robert Ritter, for example, did research on Sinti and Roma people. He mainly focused on genealogical and epidemiological studies, which contributed to developing identification and selection criteria for "Gypsies", who would then be deported to the "Gypsy camp" at Auschwitz.[27]

Granted, resistance and attempts to sabotage the many wrongs committed in the field of psychiatry during the Nazi era did exist. Even if over 50 percent of physicians were members of a National Socialist organisation, i.e. the party itself or the SA or SS, that means that almost half of all doctors were not. So doctors did have some room for manoeuvre that they could take advantage of without sanctions being imposed, and resistance did not necessarily have negative personal consequences.[28]

Indeed, some did resist, although they were too few in number, all too few. Among doctors with private practices, in particular, there were some who did not report a single case of possible hereditary disease to the public health authorities between 1934 and 1939.[29] One reason for this might have been that doctors working outside large hospitals had much more direct contact with their patients. This fact should serve as a reminder to us not to lose sight of the patients we care for, despite the demands and pressures of our everyday work. We must never allow our professional practice to be guided by ideology, but only by the wellbeing of our patients.

[25] Peiffer J (2000) Neuropathology research on 'Euthanasia' victims in two Kaiser Wilhelm Institutes [Neuropathologische Forschung an 'Euthanasie'-Opfern in zwei Kaiser-Wilhelm-Instituten]. In: Kaufmann D (ed) The Kaiser Wilhelm Society under national socialism [Die Kaiser-Wilhelm-Gesellschaft im Nationalsozialismus]. Wallstein, Göttingen, pp 151–173.

[26] Peiffer J (1997) Brain research in the shadows: examples of corruptible science during national socialism [Hirnforschung im Zwielicht: Beispiele verführbarer Wissenschaft aus der Zeit des Nationalsozialismus]. Matthiesen, Husum; Reports of the commission to inspect the specimen collections in the medical facilities at the University of Tübingen with regard to the victims of national socialism [Berichte der Kommission zur Überprüfung der Präparatesammlungen in den medizinischen Einrichtungen der Universität Tübingen im Hinblick auf Opfer des Nationalsozialismus], issued by the president of the University of Tübingen, Tübingen, 1990; Seidelman W (2010) Academic medicine during the Nazi period: The implications of creating awareness of professional responsibility today. In: Rubenfeld S (ed) Medicine after the Holocaust. Palgrave, New York, pp 29–36.

[27] Zimmermann M (2007) From education to extermination: Policy towards and research on gypsies in 20th century Europe [Zwischen Erziehung und Vernichtung: Zigeunerpolitik und Zigeunerforschung im Europa des 20. Jahrhunderts]. F. Steiner, Stuttgart, specifically the contributions by A. Cottebrune, M. Luchterhandt and E. Rosenhaft.

[28] Lifton RJ (1993) Physicians in the Third Reich [Ärzte im Dritten Reich]. Klett-Cotta, Stuttgart, p 93ff; Klee E, p 223 ff; Roelcke V (2010) Medicine during the Nazi period: Historical facts and some implications for teaching medical ethics and professionalism. In: Rubenfeld S (ed) Medicine after the Holocaust. Palgrave, New York, pp 17–28.

[29] Ley A (2004) Forced sterilisation and the medical community: the background to and objectives of physicians' actions [Zwangssterilisation und Ärzteschaft: Hintergründe und Ziele ärztlichen Handelns]. Campus, Frankfurt/M., pp 230–303.

Die Körper und einzelne Präparate der vielen Getöteten waren für Forschungszwecke begehrt und anhand dieser Präparate gewonnene Forschungsergebnisse wurden noch nach dem Krieg veröffentlicht. Im Kaiser-Wilhelm-Institut für Hirnforschung in Berlin-Buch wurden die Gehirne von mindestens 295 „Euthanasie"-Opfern zur Forschung verwendet.[25] Und noch bis in die Gegenwart hinein gab es einen fast sorglosen Umgang mit Präparaten getöteter Patientinnen und Patienten.[26]

Außerhalb psychiatrischer Institutionen fand Forschung beispielsweise des Tübinger Psychiaters Robert Ritter an Sinti und Roma statt. Diese Forschung war eine weitgehend genealogisch-epidemiologische und trug dazu bei, Identifizierungs- und Selektionskriterien für sog. „Zigeuner" zu finden, die dann in das „Zigeunerlager" im KZ Auschwitz deportiert wurden.[27]

Gegen all dieses Unrecht in der Psychiatrie zur Zeit des Nationalsozialismus hat es durchaus Widerstand gegeben und Sabotage. Über 50% der Mediziner waren Mitglied einer nationalsozialistischen Organisation, der NSDAP, SA oder SS. Das heißt aber auch, dass fast die Hälfte der Ärzte gerade nicht Mitglied war. Es gab also durchaus Handlungsspielräume, die genutzt werden konnten, ohne Sanktionen nach sich zu ziehen. Widerstand hatte nicht immer negative, persönliche Konsequenzen.[28]

Einige haben Widerstand geleistet. Aber es waren insgesamt nur wenige, viel zu wenige. Vor allem unter niedergelassenen Ärzten gab es solche, die zwischen 1934 und 1939 keine einzige Anzeige auf Vorliegen von möglichen Erberkrankungen bei den zuständigen Amtsärzten und Gesundheitsämtern erstatteten.[29] Ein Grund könnte darin liegen, dass dort, außerhalb der großen Kliniken, der Kontakt zu den Patientinnen und Patienten direkter war, unmittelbarer. Auch das ist heute eine Mahnung an uns, dass wir im Arbeitsalltag die Patientinnen und Patienten nicht aus dem Blick verlieren, die wir betreuen und begleiten. Nur sie sind die Richtschnur unseres ärztlichen Handelns, nicht die Ideologie einer Gesellschaft. Nur die einzelnen Menschen.

[25] Peiffer J (2000) Neuropathologische Forschung an „Euthanasie"-Opfern in zwei Kaiser-Wilhelm-Instituten. In: Kaufmann D (Hrsg) Die Kaiser-Wilhelm-Gesellschaft im Nationalsozialismus. Wallstein, Göttingen, S 151–173.

[26] Peiffer J (1997) Hirnforschung im Zwielicht: Beispiele verführbarer Wissenschaft aus der Zeit des Nationalsozialismus. Matthiesen, Husum; Berichte der Kommission zur Überprüfung der Präparatesammlungen in den medizinischen Einrichtungen der Universität Tübingen im Hinblick auf Opfer des Nationalsozialismus, hrsg. vom Präsidenten der Universität Tübingen, Tübingen 1990; Seidelman W (2010) Academic medicine during the Nazi period: The implications of creating awareness of professional responsibility today. In: Rubenfeld S (Hrsg) Medicine after the Holocaust. Palgrave, New York, S 29–36.

[27] Zimmermann M (2007) Zwischen Erziehung und Vernichtung: Zigeunerpolitik und Zigeunerforschung im Europa des 20. Jahrhunderts. F. Steiner, Stuttgart, darin die Beiträge von A. Cottebrune, M. Luchterhandt und E. Rosenhaft.

[28] Lifton RJ (1993) Ärzte im Dritten Reich. Klett-Cotta, Stuttgart, S 93ff; Klee E, S 223ff; Roelcke V (2010) Medicine during the Nazi period: Historical facts and some implications for teaching medical ethics and professionalism. In: Rubenfeld S (Hrsg) Medicine after the Holocaust. Palgrave, New York, S 17–28.

[29] Ley A (2004) Zwangssterilisation und Ärzteschaft: Hintergründe und Ziele ärztlichen Handelns. Campus, Frankfurt/M., S 230–303.

Human dignity is always the dignity of the individual human being. No law may ever be allowed to disregard this. In 1946 Gustav Radbruch described the conflict between law and justice. In principle, the law takes precedence over justice "unless the extent to which a positive law contradicts justice is so intolerable that it must yield to justice as 'wrongful law'. [...] When justice is not even aspired to and when equality, the very essence of justice, is deliberately flouted when drafting a positive law, such law is not only 'wrongful', it is completely devoid of legality".[30]

After the war ended, much the same occurred in the field of psychiatry as in many other areas of German society – collective denial. Neither psychiatric societies nor individual psychiatrists – with very few exceptions, such as Gerhard Schmidt and Werner Leibbrand – owned up to what had happened. This is a fact that leaves us utterly incredulous and deeply ashamed today.

---

30 Radbruch G (1946) Legal injustice and justice beyond the law [Gesetzliches Unrecht und übergesetzliches Recht]. Süddeutsche Juristenzeitung 1: 105–108, specifically p 107.

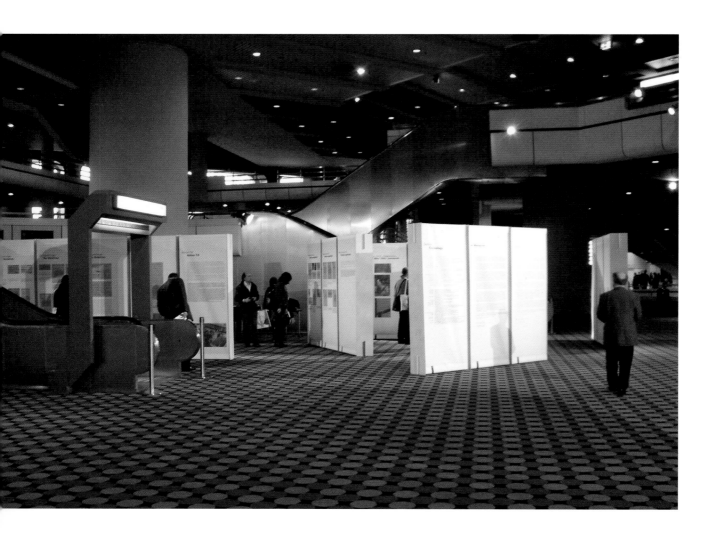

Die Menschenwürde ist immer die Würde des einzelnen Menschen. Dies zu missachten darf uns kein Gesetz anleiten. Gustav Radbruch beschrieb 1946 den Konfliktfall zwischen Recht und Gerechtigkeit: Das gesetzte Recht hat prinzipiell den Vorrang vor der Gerechtigkeit, „es sei denn, daß der Widerspruch des positiven Gesetzes zur Gerechtigkeit ein so unerträgliches Maß erreicht, daß das Gesetz als ‚unrichtiges Recht' der Gerechtigkeit zu weichen hat. (…) Wo Gerechtigkeit nicht einmal erstrebt wird, wo die Gleichheit, die den Kern der Gerechtigkeit ausmacht, bei der Setzung positiven Rechts bewußt verleugnet wurde, da ist das Gesetz nicht etwa nur ‚unrichtiges Recht', vielmehr entbehrt es überhaupt der Rechtsnatur".[30]

Nach dem Krieg geschah, was auch in vielen anderen Bereichen in Deutschland geschah. Es wurde verdrängt. Die psychiatrischen Fachgesellschaften wie die Psychiater – mit einigen, ganz wenigen Ausnahmen wie Gerhard Schmidt oder Werner Leibbrand – haben sich nicht zu dem bekannt, was geschehen ist. Dafür empfinden wir heute Scham und sind fassungslos.

---

[30] Radbruch G (1946) Gesetzliches Unrecht und übergesetzliches Recht. Süddeutsche Juristenzeitung 1: 105–108, dort S 107.

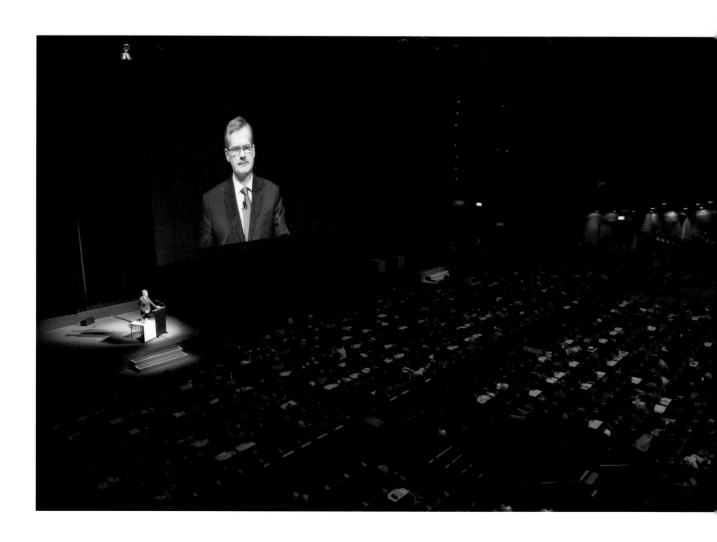

The story of Professor Werner Heyde, who has already been mentioned, is particularly mindboggling.[31] Heyde was the medical director of the "T4 program", and an arrest warrant was issued for him after the war. And yet from 1950 to 1959 he enjoyed a second career as a court-appointed medical expert in Schleswig-Holstein. Although he went by the name of Dr. Fritz Sawade, there were those in the medical and legal professions who were aware of his real identity, yet did not expose him. And many others, both within our field and beyond, knew about it.

At the same time, early attempts to shed light on the wrongs committed by physicians during the Nazi era were impeded and thwarted. When Alexander Mitscherlich and Fred Mielke released their book *Das Diktat der Menschenverachtung* [The Dictate of Contempt for Human Life],[32] which documented the trials of medical doctors in Nuremberg in 1947, many doctors protested because they were worried that the reputation of their profession would be tarnished. When the duo's second book *Wissenschaft ohne Menschlichkeit*[33] [Science without Humanity], was published in 1949, it was ignored.

---

[31] Cf. Godau-Schüttke K-D (2010) The Heyde/Sawade affair [Die Heyde/Sawade-Affäre], 3rd edition. Nomos, Baden-Baden.

[32] Mitscherlich A, Mielke F (1947) The dictate of contempt for human life: a documentation [Das Diktat der Menschenverachtung: eine Dokumentation]. Lambert Schneider, Heidelberg.

[33] First published under the title "Science without humanity" [Wissenschaft ohne Menschlichkeit]. Lambert Schneider, Heidelberg, 1949; from 1960 on under the title "Medicine without humanity: documents on the Nuremberg doctors' trials" [Medizin ohne Menschlichkeit: Dokumente des Nürnberger Ärzteprozesses]. S. Fischer-Verlag, Frankfurt/M., 16th edition, 2004.

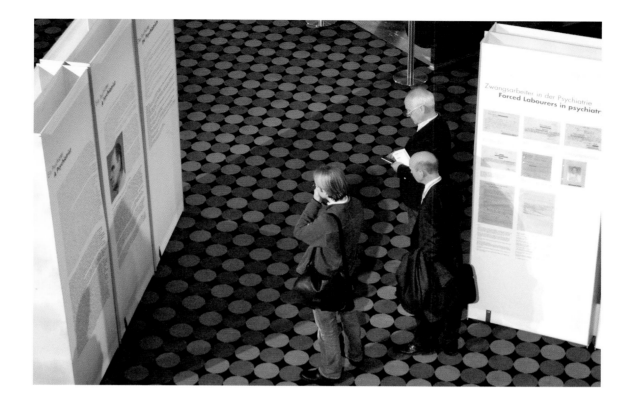

Unfassbar ist bis heute die Geschichte des bereits erwähnten Professors Werner Heyde.[31] Er war der medizinische Leiter der „T4"-Aktion. Nach dem Krieg wurde er per Haftbefehl gesucht und machte unter dem Namen Dr. med. Fritz Sawade von 1950 bis 1959 dennoch eine zweite Karriere als Gerichtsgutachter in Schleswig-Holstein. Er wurde von Ärzten und Juristen gedeckt, die über seine wahre Identität informiert waren. Und viele andere, denen seine Doppelidentität ebenso bekannt war, unternahmen nichts – und es war bekannt, innerhalb und außerhalb unseres Faches.

Zugleich wurden frühe Versuche der Aufklärung verhindert und erschwert. Viele Ärzte protestierten, weil sie um ihre Standesehre besorgt waren, als Alexander Mitscherlich und Fred Mielke 1947 ihre Dokumentation „Das Diktat der Menschenverachtung"[32] zum Nürnberger Ärzteprozess veröffentlichten. Eine zweite Dokumentation von 1949, „Wissenschaft ohne Menschlichkeit"[33], wurde totgeschwiegen.

---

[31] Vgl. Godau-Schüttke K-D (2010) Die Heyde/Sawade-Affäre, 3. Auflage. Nomos, Baden-Baden.

[32] Mitscherlich A, Mielke F (Hrsg) (1947) Das Diktat der Menschenverachtung: eine Dokumentation. Lambert Schneider, Heidelberg.

[33] Erstveröffentlichung unter dem Titel „Wissenschaft ohne Menschlichkeit", Lambert Schneider, Heidelberg, 1949, ab 1960 unter dem Titel „Medizin ohne Menschlichkeit: Dokumente des Nürnberger Ärzteprozesses". S. Fischer-Verlag, Frankfurt/M. (16. Auflage), 2004.

Professor Gerhard Schmidt, the former director of the psychiatric clinic in Lübeck, gave a radio talk about the crimes committed against the mentally ill and the mentally disabled as early as 20 November 1945 – yet he was unable to find a publisher for his book manuscript on the topic for 20 years, despite numerous attempts.[34] I read the book many years ago, and it had a profound impact on me. But many psychiatrists in post-war Germany were afraid that publicising the details of these crimes would endanger efforts to rebuild their profession and damage its reputation, which they saw still positive at the time. A grievously misguided view, for the scientific community thus failed to acknowledge its responsibility. The German Psychiatric Association honoured Professor Schmidt for his life's work by presenting him with its Wilhelm Griesinger Medal in 1986, the first year it was awarded. One of our organisation's prouder moments, even if it came far too late and has sadly been almost forgotten.

And what about official legislation? The German federal government enacted the *Bundesgesetz zur Entschädigung für Opfer der nationalsozialistischen Verfolgung* or BEG [Federal Indemnification Law] in 1956, which provided for the indemnification of victims of Nazi persecution and came into force with retroactive effect. After some revisions, the *BEG-Schlussgesetz* [BEG – Final Law] was passed in 1965. Thus all victims who had suffered persecution under the Nazi regime due to their race, religion, or political views could file a claim for indemnification by 1969. However, the law did not apply to those who had been forcibly sterilised or to the families of victims of the "euthanasia", since – it was argued – they had not been persecuted due to their race[35] – a further humiliation of the victims, and still we did not speak out.

---

[34] Schmidt G (1965) Selection in the psychiatric hospital 1939–1945 [Selektion in der Heilanstalt 1939–1945]. Evangelisches Verlagswerk, Stuttgart.

[35] Cf. written report of the Restitution Committee, Bundestag printed paper 2382, pp 12f and p 57; for a good overview on this and the following cf. Surmann R (2005) What is typical Nazi injustice? The denial of compensation for victims of forced sterilisation and 'Euthanasia' [Was ist typisches NS-Unrecht? Die verweigerte Entschädigung für Zwangssterilisierte und 'Euthanasie'-Geschädigte]. In: Hamm M (ed) Unworthy of living – destroyed life. Forced sterilisation and Euthanasia [Lebensunwert – zerstörte Leben. Zwangssterilisation und Euthanasie]. VAS-Verlag, Frankfurt/M., pp 198–211; Scheulen A (2005) The legal status and development of the 1934 sterilisation law [Zur Rechtslage und Rechtsentwicklung des Erbgesundheitsgesetzes 1934]. In: Hamm M (ed) Unworthy of living – destroyed life. Forced sterilisation and Euthanasia [Lebensunwert – zerstörte Leben. Zwangssterilisation und Euthanasie]. VAS-Verlag, Frankfurt/M., pp 212–219.

Professor Gerhard Schmidt, ehemaliger Direktor der Nervenklinik Lübeck, hielt schon am 20. November 1945 einen Rundfunkvortrag über die Verbrechen an psychisch Kranken und geistig Behinderten – aber sein Buchmanuskript darüber fand trotz vieler Versuche 20 Jahre lang keinen Verleger.[34] Ich hatte es vor vielen Jahren gelesen, ein Buch, das mich außerordentlich stark geprägt hat. Psychiater des Nachkriegsdeutschlands aber fürchteten, dem Wiederaufbau und dem – noch immer – guten Ruf der deutschen Psychiater insgesamt mit der Veröffentlichung der Einzelheiten der Verbrechen einen schlechten Dienst zu erweisen, was eine falsche, eine fatale Sichtweise war, ein Versagen der wissenschaftlichen Gemeinschaft, sich zu der eigenen Verantwortung zu bekennen. 1986 erhielt Professor Schmidt für sein Lebenswerk die in jenem Jahr erstmals vergebene Wilhelm-Griesinger-Medaille der Deutschen Gesellschaft für Psychiatrie und Nervenheilkunde. Eine fast vergessene, viel zu späte und seltene Sternstunde unserer Gesellschaft.

Und die Politik? 1956 wurde rückwirkend das Bundesgesetz zur Entschädigung für Opfer der nationalsozialistischen Verfolgung verabschiedet. 1965 wurde es zum BEG-Schlussgesetz erweitert. So konnten bis 1969 alle Opfer, die aus rassischen, religiösen oder politischen Gründe verfolgt worden waren, einen Anspruch auf Entschädigung anmelden – nicht aber die Zwangssterilisierten oder die Familien von Euthanasieopfern, weil sie nicht aus rassischen Gründen verfolgt worden seien.[35] Auch dies eine nachträgliche Demütigung der Opfer, zu der wir geschwiegen haben.

---

[34] Schmidt G (1965) Selektion in der Heilanstalt 1939–1945. Evangelisches Verlagswerk, Stuttgart.

[35] Vgl. Schriftlicher Bericht des Ausschuss für Fragen der Wiedergutmachung, Bundestagsdrucksache 2382, S 12f und S 57; hierzu und zum Folgenden als Überblick: Surmann R (2005) Was ist typisches NS-Unrecht? Die verweigerte Entschädigung für Zwangssterilisierte und ‚Euthanasie'-Geschädigte. In: Hamm M (Hrsg) Lebensunwert – zerstörte Leben. Zwangssterilisation und Euthanasie. VAS-Verlag, Frankfurt/M., S 198–211; Scheulen A (2005) Zur Rechtslage und Rechtsentwicklung des Erbgesundheitsgesetzes 1934. In: Hamm M (Hrsg) Lebensunwert – zerstörte Leben. Zwangssterilisation und Euthanasie. VAS-Verlag, Frankfurt/M., S 212–219.

Some of the expert witnesses called on during the hearings of the West German Bundestag's Restitution Committee in the 1960s were the same psychiatrists who had justified forced sterilisations and participated in systematic murder during the Third Reich. Records of 13th April 1961 report that Werner Villinger rejected the idea of compensation payments on the contemptuous grounds that the payments might cause victims of forced sterilisation to develop "neurotic ailments and suffering that could damage not only their current well-being and [...] their ability to enjoy life, but also their ability to perform."[36]

The Law for the Prevention of Hereditarily Diseased Offspring was not suspended until 1974. Formally, though, it continued to exist. In 1988 the West German Bundestag concluded that the forced sterilisations carried out under the Law counted as Nazi injustices. Ten years later the Bundestag passed a law repealing the rulings of the genetic health courts. Yet it took the Bundestag until 2007 to finally ban the Law for the Prevention of Hereditarily Diseased Offspring[37]. The reason given was that the Law contravened the Basic Law anyway, so was effectively suspended at the time that came into force. The DGPPN supported calls to ban the Law at the time.

The Federal Indemnification Act of 1965, however, applies to this day, which means that mentally ill people who were forcibly sterilised or murdered have still not been explicitly acknowledged as victims of the Nazi regime or as victims of racial persecution. Lawmakers need to take action and change this before it is too late. Victims will not have received due recognition of their pain and suffering, which continues to this day, until the German government repeals this injustice as well.

The late 1960s and 1970s saw the first attempts to publish accounts of what happened in the field of psychiatry. Hans-Jörg Weitbrecht, Walter Ritter von Baeyer and Helmut Ehrhardt[38] all wrote on the topic, yet all three presented psychiatry itself as a victim.[39] A book commemorating the 130th anniversary of the German Association for Psychiatry and Psychotherapy in 1972 says that: "representatives of the psychiatric profession, despite their apparently far-reaching authority, never supported, endorsed or aided abuses such as 'euthanasia' ex officio. This is another reason to reject as objectively unfounded the repeated attempts to charge 'German psychiatry' with the misconduct or the crimes committed by individual psychiatrists at the time".[40]

---

[36] Minutes of the 34th session of the Restitution Committee, Thursday 13 April 1961, p 16.

[37] Plenary minutes 16/100, 100th session of the German Bundestag, Berlin, Thursday 24 May 2007.

[38] Ehrhardt HE (1965) Euthanasia and the "destruction of life unworthy of living" [Euthanasie und "Vernichtung lebensunwerten Lebens"]. F. Enke, Stuttgart; von Baeyer W (1966) The vindication of Nazi ideology in medicine with particular regard to Euthanasia [Die Bestätigung der NS-Ideologie in der Medizin unter besonderer Berücksichtigung der Euthanasie]. National socialism and the German university, Free University 1966 [Nationalsozialismus und die Deutsche Universität, Freie Universität 1966]. de Gruyter, Berlin, pp 63–75; Weitbrecht H-J (1968) Psychiatry under national socialism [Psychiatrie in der Zeit des Nationalsozialismus]. P. Hanstein, Bonn.

[39] Cf. the analysis in Roelcke V (2007) Trauma or responsibility? Memories and historiographies of Nazi psychiatry in postwar Germany. In: Sarat A, Davidovich N, Alberstein M (eds) Trauma and memory. Reading, healing, and making law. Stanford University Press, Stanford, pp 225–242.

[40] Ehrhardt HE (1972) 130 years of the German Association for Psychiatry and Psychotherapy [130 Jahre Deutsche Gesellschaft für Psychiatrie und Nervenheilkunde]. Wiesbaden, p 15.

Gutachter in den Anhörungen des Bundestagsausschusses für Wiedergutmachung in den 1960er Jahre waren zum Teil dieselben Psychiater, die im Nationalsozialismus Zwangssterilisierungen gerechtfertigt hatten und an den Tötungsaktionen beteiligt waren. Am 13. April 1961 lehnte Werner Villinger laut Protokoll Entschädigungszahlungen mit der zynischen Begründung ab, es sei die Frage, ob bei der Durchführung einer Entschädigung der Zwangssterilisierten „nicht neurotische Beschwerden und Leiden auftreten, die nicht nur das bisherige Wohlbefinden und (…) die Glücksfähigkeit dieser Menschen, sondern auch ihre Leistungsfähigkeit beeinträchtigen."[36]

Erst 1974 wurde das Erbgesundheitsgesetz außer Kraft gesetzt. Es bestand aber formal weiter. 1988 stellte der Deutsche Bundestag fest, dass die auf der Grundlage des Erbgesundheitsgesetzes vorgenommenen Zwangssterilisierungen nationalsozialistisches Unrecht waren. Zehn Jahre später beschloss der Bundestag, die Entscheidungen der Erbgesundheitsgerichte per Gesetz aufzuheben. Aber erst 2007 wurde schließlich das Gesetz zur Verhütung erbkranken Nachwuchses vom Deutschen Bundestag geächtet.[37] Es stünde im Widerspruch zum Grundgesetz und sei daher faktisch bereits bei dessen Inkrafttreten außer Kraft getreten. Die DGPPN hatte diesen Antrag zur Ächtung des Gesetzes seinerzeit unterstützt.

Weiterhin Bestand aber hat das Bundesentschädigungsgesetz von 1965. Bis heute sind die zwangssterilisierten und ermordeten psychisch kranken Menschen daher nicht explizit als Opfer des NS-Regimes und als Verfolgte aus rassischen Gründen anerkannt. Hier sollte die Politik aktiv werden, bevor es zu spät ist. Erst mit der Aufhebung auch dieses Unrechts würde das fortdauernde Leid der Opfer und ihr Schicksal auch von Seiten des deutschen Staates angemessen gewürdigt.

Mit Bezug auf die Psychiatrie gab es in den späten 1960er und 1970er Jahren erste vereinzelte Publikationen, die Vorgänge darzustellen, so von Hans-Jörg Weitbrecht, Walter Ritter von Baeyer oder Helmut Ehrhardt.[38] Aber alle drei haben die Psychiatrie als Opfer dargestellt.[39] In einem Buch zur 130-jährigen Geschichte der Deutsche Gesellschaft für Psychiatrie und Nervenheilkunde von 1972 heißt es, „daß die damalige Vertretung der Psychiater, trotz ihrer scheinbar weitreichenden Befugnisse, ex officio niemals Aktionen wie die ‚Euthanasie' gedeckt, befürwortet oder gefördert hat. Auch deswegen sind die wiederholten Versuche, das Fehlverhalten oder die Verbrechen einzelner Psychiater dieser Zeit ‚der deutschen Psychiatrie' anzulasten, als objektiv unbegründet zurückzuweisen".[40]

---

[36] Protokoll zur 34. Sitzung des Ausschusses für Wiedergutmachung, Donnerstag, den 13. April 1961, S 16.

[37] Plenarprotokoll 16/100, 100. Sitzung des Deutschen Bundestages, Berlin, Donnerstag, den 24. Mai 2007.

[38] Ehrhardt HE (1965) Euthanasie und „Vernichtung lebensunwerten Lebens". F. Enke, Stuttgart; von Baeyer W (1966) „Die Bestätigung der NS-Ideologie in der Medizin unter besonderer Berücksichtigung der Euthanasie". In: Nationalsozialismus und die Deutsche Universität, Freie Universität 1966. de Gruyter, Berlin, S 63–75; Weitbrecht H-J (1968) Psychiatrie in der Zeit des Nationalsozialismus. P. Hanstein, Bonn.

[39] Vgl. dazu die Analyse in Roelcke V (2007) Trauma or responsibility? Memories and historiographies of Nazi psychiatry in postwar Germany. In: Sarat A, Davidovich N, Alberstein M (Hrsg) Trauma and memory. Reading, healing, and making law. Stanford University Press, Stanford, S 225–242.

[40] Ehrhardt HE (1972) 130 Jahre Deutsche Gesellschaft für Psychiatrie und Nervenheilkunde. Steiner, Wiesbaden, S 15.

This was written by Helmut Ehrhardt, President of the DGPN from 1970 to 1972, who himself had been a member of the NSDAP and who had written reports endorsing forced sterilisation. As late as the hearings for the Federal Indemnification Act in the West German Bundestag in 1961, he said that the "actual content"[41] of the Law for the Prevention of Hereditarily Diseased Offspring "was certainly not an invention of the Nazi regime, but rather something that in its essence reflected and still reflects current scientific conviction".[42] This further mocks and degrades victims.

It is true that the association never officially endorsed killing patients. However, it is also true that it never officially condemned the practice either. There was never a single word of apology or reprimand.

And yet, with just a few exceptions, it appears that the overwhelming majority of German psychiatrists and members of our association, whether researchers, academics or practitioners, took part in planning, implementing and creating scientific legitimacy for sterilisation and murder.[43]

Research into German psychiatry under National Socialism only began in earnest in the early 1980s.[44] The main contributions from psychiatrists came from Klaus Dörner – who began in 1969 and produced a series of publications in the 1980s – Asmus Finzen and Joachim-Ernst Meyer. Among the historians were Gerhard Baader, Dirk Blasius and Hans-Walter Schmuhl. In 1983 Ernst Klee published his shocking book, '"Euthanasia" in the Nazi State', which I read at the time in stunned disbelief. So this was another book that deeply affected me.

During an anniversary congress held under the presidency of Uwe Henrik Peters in Cologne in 1992 – when the name of the association was changed to DGPPN – the General Meeting passed a resolution in which the association reinforced "its feelings of revulsion and sorrow about the holocaust of the mentally ill, Jews and other victims of persecution." Back then there was no mention of the institutional and personal guilt of psychiatrists and their representative organisation. However, it was a clear message that needed to be articulated.

---

[41] German Bundestag, minutes of the 34th session of the Restitution Committee, Thursday 13 April 1961, top of p 25.

[42] Ibid, bottom of page.

[43] Cf. Meyer-Lindenberg J (1991) The Holocaust and German Psychiatry. Br J Psychiatry 159: 7–12, especially p 9; Roelcke V (2010) Psychiatry under national socialism. Historical findings, implications for current ethical debates [Psychiatrie im Nationalsozialismus. Historische Kenntnisse, Implikationen für aktuelle ethische Debatten]. Nervenarzt 81: 1317–1325.

[44] For more on the history of the psychiatric profession coming to terms with its past cf. Roelcke, Trauma or responsibility (note 39).

Autor war der Präsident der DGPN der Jahre 1970–1972, Helmut Ehrhardt, der selbst Mitglied der NSDAP gewesen war und Gutachten erstellt hatte, in denen er die Zwangssterilisierungen befürwortete. Noch in der Anhörung zum Bundesentschädigungsgesetz im Deutschen Bundestag im Jahr 1961 betonte er, dass der „materielle Gehalt"[41] des Erbgesundheitsgesetzes „sicher nicht eine nationalsozialistische Erfindung ist, sondern in seinem Kerngehalt wirklich der damaligen und auch der heutigen wissenschaftlichen Überzeugung entspricht".[42] Eine erneute Verhöhnung und Erniedrigung der Opfer.

Richtig ist, dass es keine offizielle befürwortende Stellungnahme der psychiatrischen Fachgesellschaft zu den Krankentötungen gab. Richtig ist aber auch, dass es keine Stellungnahme dagegen gab – kein Wort, keine Entschuldigung, keine Mahnung.

Bis auf wenige Einzelne beteiligte sich damals offensichtlich die große Mehrheit der deutschen Psychiater und Mitglieder unserer Fachgesellschaft bis hin zu deren Vorstand in Forschung, Wissenschaft und Praxis an der Planung, Durchführung und wissenschaftlichen Legitimierung von Selektion, Sterilisation und Tötung.[43]

Ernsthaft begann die Erforschung der Geschichte der Psychiatrie in Deutschland in der Zeit des Nationalsozialismus seit etwa Anfang der 1980er Jahre.[44] Als Psychiater waren dies wesentlich Klaus Dörner – erstmals 1969, dann mit mehreren Publikationen in den 1980er Jahren –, Asmus Finzen und Joachim-Ernst Meyer. Unter den Historikern sind Gerhard Baader, Dirk Blasius und Hans Walter Schmuhl zu nennen. Und 1983 erschien das aufrüttelnde Buch von Ernst Klee „,Euthanasie' im NS-Staat", das ich damals ganz ungläubig und fassungslos gelesen hatte. Auch dies ein Buch, das mich außerordentlich betroffen machte.

Im Rahmen des sog. Jubiläumskongresses unter der Präsidentschaft von Uwe Henrik Peters, 1992 in Köln – dort ist die Gesellschaft in die DGPPN umbenannt worden –, wurde in der Mitgliederversammlung eine Resolution verabschiedet, in der die Gesellschaft „ihren Abscheu und ihre Trauer im Rückblick auf den Holocaust an Geisteskranken, Juden und anderen verfolgten Menschen" bekräftigt. Damals war noch nicht von der institutionellen und persönlichen Schuld und Verstrickung der Psychiater und ihrer Fachgesellschaft die Rede. Aber es waren dennoch deutliche, notwendige Worte.

---

[41] Deutscher Bundestag, Protokoll 34. Sitzung des Ausschusses für Wiedergutmachung, Donnerstag, den 13. April 1961, S 25 oben.

[42] Ebd, unten.

[43] Vgl. Meyer-Lindenberg J (1991) The Holocaust and German Psychiatry. Br J Psychiatry 159: 7–12, dort S 9; Roelcke V (2010) Psychiatrie im Nationalsozialismus. Historische Kenntnisse, Implikationen für aktuelle ethische Debatten. Nervenarzt 81: 1317–1325.

[44] Zur Geschichte der Aufarbeitung, vgl. Roelcke, Trauma or responsibility (Fußnote 39).

During this year's congress we are showing a revised and updated version of the *In Memoriam* exhibition[45], which drew large international audiences when it was first shown in 1999 at the World Congress of Psychiatry in Hamburg. A series of symposia accompanied the exhibition. The decision by the World Psychiatric Association to select Germany and the DGPPN as the hosts of the World Congress was a conciliatory gesture from the international psychiatric community – and it presented us with the solemn duty to begin commemorating the victims and to make serious efforts to come to terms with the history of our profession.

Over the past two years the DGPPN has held a series of in-depth discussions about how to deal with its own history. These talks were not controversial; they were conducted by mutual agreement. As a result of the talks, we amended the DGPPN's Articles of Association exactly one year ago. The first paragraph now reads:

"The DGPPN recognises that it bears a special responsibility to protect the dignity and rights of people suffering from mental illness. This responsibility is the result of its predecessors' involvement in the crimes of National Socialism, in killing and forcibly sterilising hundreds of thousands of patients."

Another outcome of the discussions was that, early this year, the DGPPN Executive Committee established an international commission to address the actions of the predecessor associations that existed during the "Third Reich". The commission is made up of four renowned historians of medicine and science: the chairman, Professor Roelcke from Gießen, Professor Sachse from Vienna, Professor Schmiedebach from Hamburg, and Professor Weindling from Oxford. The commission makes its decisions independently of the DGPPN, as we realise how important complete transparency is in this type of work. We are extremely grateful to the members of the commission for helping us in our efforts to come to terms with our past.

The commission is overseeing the DGPPN-initiated and financed research projects involving Professor Schmuhl and Professor Zalashik. They aim to shed light on the extent to which the DGPPN's predecessor organisations and their representatives were involved in the "euthanasia" programme, in forced sterilisations of mentally ill patients and in other crimes between 1933 and 1945.

---

[45] von Cranach M, Schneider F (2010) In Memoriam. Remembrance and responsibility. Exhibition catalogue. Springer, Berlin.

Während des diesjährigen Kongresses zeigen wir überarbeitet und aktualisiert die Ausstellung „In Memoriam", die erstmals auf dem Weltkongress der World Psychiatric Association 1999 in Hamburg einer großen, internationalen Öffentlichkeit gezeigt wurde.[45] Symposien begleiteten die Ausstellung. Dass damals die internationale Entscheidung auf Deutschland als Gastgeberland des Weltkongresses mit der DGPPN als gastgebender Fachgesellschaft fiel, war ein versöhnliches Zeichen der psychiatrischen Weltgemeinschaft – und es war eine große Verpflichtung, mit dem Gedenken an die Opfer und der Auseinandersetzung unserer fachspezifischen Vergangenheit Ernst zu machen.

In den vergangenen knapp zwei Jahren hat innerhalb der DGPPN ein intensiver Diskussionsprozess stattgefunden, wie mit der eigenen Geschichte umgegangen werden soll. Diese Diskussionen wurden nicht kontrovers, sondern sehr einvernehmlich geführt. Vor genau einem Jahr schließlich wurde die Satzung der DGPPN ergänzt. Es heißt nun dort im ersten Paragrafen:

„Die DGPPN ist sich ihrer besonderen Verantwortung um die Würde und Rechte der psychisch Kranken bewusst, die ihr aus der Beteiligung ihrer Vorläuferorganisationen an den Verbrechen des Nationalsozialismus, an massenhaften Krankenmorden und Zwangssterilisationen erwachsen."

Als weitere Konsequenz dieses Diskussionsprozesses wurde zu Beginn dieses Jahres vom Vorstand der DGPPN eine internationale Kommission zur Aufarbeitung der Geschichte der Vorläufergesellschaften in der Zeit des Nationalsozialismus eingerichtet. Sie ist mit vier namhaften Medizin- und Wissenschaftshistorikern besetzt, dem Vorsitzenden Professor Roelcke aus Gießen, Frau Professor Sachse aus Wien, Herrn Professor Schmiedebach aus Hamburg und Herrn Professor Weindling aus Oxford. Die Kommission ist in ihren Entscheidungen unabhängig von der DGPPN, da wir eine vollständige Transparenz gerade auch dieser Arbeit wollen. Den Mitgliedern der Kommission sind wir für die Unterstützung und Hilfe bei der Aufklärung unserer eigenen Vergangenheit außerordentlich dankbar.

Die Kommission begleitet die von der Fachgesellschaft initiierten und finanzierten Forschungsprojekte, an denen Professor Schmuhl und Frau Professor Zalashik arbeiten. Sie sollen klären, inwieweit die Vorläuferorganisationen der DGPPN und deren Repräsentanten bei dem sog. Euthanasieprogramm, der Zwangssterilisierung psychisch Kranker, der Vertreibung jüdischer und politisch missliebiger Psychiater und anderen Verbrechen in der Zeit zwischen 1933 und 1945 beteiligt waren.

---

[45] von Cranach M, Schneider F (2010) In Memoriam. Erinnerung und Verantwortung. Ausstellungskatalog. Springer, Berlin.

The final report is due to be presented in just under two years, after which a second phase will begin the equally long-overdue task of addressing the post-war period. It will explore the consequences of the terrible crimes perpetrated under the Nazis, uncover who was involved, and reveal what lessons were learned and when. This will replace the speculation surrounding this period with solid facts.

"Mentally dead", "human ballast", "life unworthy of living" – these are not easy words to say. They are deeply upsetting and disturbing – and, in light of the fact that psychiatrists were actively involved in "Gleichschaltung", forced sterilisation and murder, they fill us with shame, anger and the greatest sorrow.

Our shame and regret are also rooted in the fact that it has taken this association, of which I am President today, 70 years to make a systematic effort to come to terms with its past and the history of its predecessors under National Socialism, and – irrespective of the historical facts that may come to light – to ask for forgiveness from the victims of forced migration, forced sterilisation, human experiments and murder.

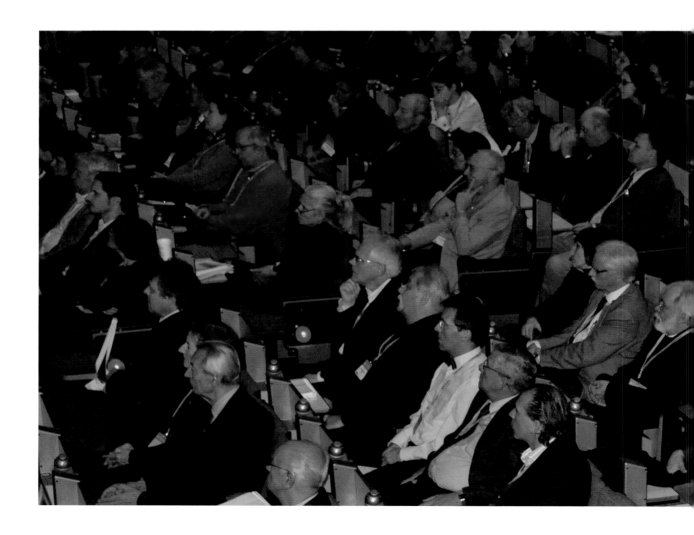

Der Abschlussbericht soll in knapp zwei Jahren vorgelegt werden, um dann in einer zweiten Arbeitsphase die ebenso fällige Aufarbeitung der Zeit nach dem zweiten Weltkrieg zu untersuchen. Auch dies ist wichtig: Welche Konsequenzen ergaben sich, welche Personen waren beteiligt, welche Lehren wurden wann aus den schrecklichen Taten im sog. „Dritten Reich" gezogen? Darüber ahnen wir mehr, als wir mit Sicherheit zu sagen wissen.

„Geistiger Tod", „Ballastexistenzen", „lebensunwertes Leben", all diese Worte gehen nur sehr schwer über die Lippen. Sie erschüttern und verstören zutiefst – und im Wissen um die aktive Beteiligung von Psychiatern an Gleichschaltung, Zwangssterilisierung und Mord erfüllen sie uns mit Scham, Zorn und großer Trauer.

Scham und Trauer auch darüber, dass erst jetzt, 70 Jahre nach den Taten, die Organisation, als deren Präsident ich hier zu Ihnen spreche, beginnt, sich systematisch mit ihrer Vergangenheit und der Geschichte ihrer Vorgängerorganisationen in der Zeit des Nationalsozialismus zu befassen, aufzuarbeiten, und – unabhängig von allen noch zu erhebenden historischen Details – bei den Opfern von Zwangsemigration, Zwangssterilisierung, Zwangsforschung und Ermordung, um Entschuldigung zu bitten.

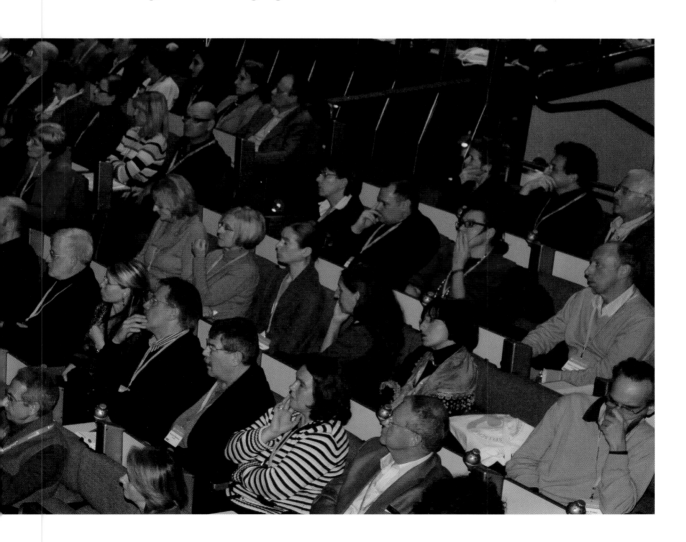

In the name of the German Association for Psychiatry and Psychotherapy, I ask you, the victims and relatives of the victims, for forgiveness for the pain and injustice you suffered in the name of German psychiatry and at the hands of German psychiatrists under National Socialism, and for the silence, trivialisation and denial that for far too long characterised psychiatry in post-war Germany.

Many of the victims, even those who were not killed, and their families are no longer with us today. For them, this request comes too late. But perhaps it is not too late for the survivors and for the victims' descendants – some of whom are with us here today – for mentally ill people everywhere and for today's psychiatrists and the DGPPN itself.

We cannot undo pain, injustice and death. But we can learn lessons, and we have learned a great many – in the psychiatry profession, in medicine as a whole, and in politics and society. And we can commemorate the victims by coming together to advocate humane, patient-oriented psychiatry and by working together to fight the stigmatisation and marginalisation of mentally ill people.

As psychiatrists, we must not pass value judgements on people. We teach, research, treat, support and cure. When we speak of the inviolability of human dignity, we mean the dignity of each and every individual, and no law or research objective must ever cause us to disregard this again.

We have learned important lessons from our failures. This offers hope for current debates on medical ethics, which, given their focus on topics such as preimplantation genetic diagnosis and assisted suicide, risk descending all too quickly into questions of the "value" of a human life. These discussions will always be murky, but I believe that my goal and the goal of the DGPPN as a whole is perfectly clear – we must ensure we provide humane medical care, contribute to a more benign future, and respect the dignity of every single individual.

Ladies and gentlemen, thank you for your attention.

The original German text of this speech was unanimously adopted by the Executive Board of the DGPPN as an Association Document on 23 November 2010. We are very grateful to Carsten Burfeind, MA, (Berlin) and Prof. Dr. Volker Roelcke (Gießen) for their comments and suggestions.

Im Namen der Deutschen Gesellschaft für Psychiatrie, Psychotherapie und Nervenheilkunde bitte ich Sie, die Opfer und deren Angehörige, um Verzeihung für das Leid und das Unrecht, das Ihnen in der Zeit des Nationalsozialismus im Namen der deutschen Psychiatrie und von deutschen Psychiaterinnen und Psychiatern angetan wurde, und für das viel zu lange Schweigen, Verharmlosen und Verdrängen der deutschen Psychiatrie in der Zeit danach.

Viele Opfer, auch diejenigen, die nicht getötet wurden und deren Angehörige, leben heute nicht mehr. Insofern kommt diese Bitte zu spät. Sie kommt aber vielleicht noch nicht zu spät für die Lebenden und die Nachfahren, einige sind heute unter uns, und für alle psychisch kranken Menschen heute und für die heutigen Psychiaterinnen und Psychiater und die DGPPN selbst.

Leid und Unrecht, schon gar nicht der Tod, können ungeschehen gemacht werden. Aber wir können lernen – und wir haben viel gelernt, die Psychiatrie ebenso wie die gesamte Medizin, Politik und Gesellschaft. Und wir können gemeinsam für eine humane, menschliche, am einzelnen Menschen orientierte Psychiatrie eintreten und arbeiten, kämpfen gegen die Stigmatisierung und Ausgrenzung psychisch Kranker, im steten Gedenken an die Opfer.

Wir Psychiaterinnen und Psychiater sollen keine Werturteile über Menschen fällen, wir lehren, forschen, behandeln, begleiten und heilen. Die unantastbare Menschenwürde ist immer die Würde des einzelnen Menschen und kein Gesetz und kein Forschungsziel dürfen uns dazu anleiten, diese zu missachten.

Wir haben gelernt, gerade auch aus dem Versagen heraus. Das stimmt hoffnungsvoll in den aktuellen medizinethischen Diskussionen, bei denen es nur zu schnell auch um den „Wert" oder „Unwert" von Menschen geht, wie denen zur Präimplantationsdiagnostik oder zur Sterbehilfe. Diese Diskussionen bleiben schwierig – aber das Ziel ist für mich, ist für die DGPPN ganz klar: Arbeiten wir für eine humane Medizin, eine menschenwürdige Zukunft und für die Achtung der Würde aller Menschen.

Sehr geehrte Damen und Herren, ich danke Ihnen für Ihre Aufmerksamkeit.

Diese Rede wurde von dem Vorstand der DGPPN am 23. November 2010 als Dokument der Gesellschaft einstimmig verabschiedet. Wir danken Carsten Burfeind, M.A., (Berlin) und Prof. Dr. Volker Roelcke (Gießen) sehr für ihre Hinweise und Kommentare.

Speech of Prof. Dr. Ephraim Bental, Haifa, Son of an Emigrated Neuropsychiatrist

Professor Schneider, Ladies and Gentlemen, Colleagues!

I am the son of a neuropsychiatrist who was forced to abandon a successful medical career in Germany all of a sudden in 1933 in the wake of the Nazi race laws. I have been full of anticipation about speaking to you at this plenary session. The commemorative event which you all are taking part in is an important milestone in efforts to come to terms with the history of German psychiatry.

Unfortunately, I am unable to attend the conference in person for health reasons, so I have to speak to you via video. I too am a neuropsychiatrist, and my talk is dedicated to the memory of my father, Dr. Kurt Blumenthal-Bental, and all the psychiatrists who were forced to suddenly give up successful medical careers and lives in Germany after 1933, to move to Palestine and rebuild their professions and lives under extremely difficult conditions.

Over 40 psychiatrists left for Palestine/Israel in those days. Many of them had held leading positions in Germany.

My father, Dr. Kurt Blumenthal, (who changed his last name to Bental in Israel in 1949 to sound more Hebrew), was born in Berlin in 1893. He was raised in the spirit of Jewish assimilation, Liberalism and the Enlightenment, which then had pervaded Europe since the early 19th century, and he received a classical German education that included Greek, Latin and French as well as thorough exposure to German and European literature and poetry. He began to study medicine in Berlin in 1912, breaking off his studies to serve as a medical officer in the First World War.

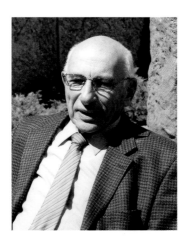

⊗ Rede von Prof. Dr. Ephraim Bental, Haifa, Sohn eines emigrierten Psychiaters

Sehr geehrter Herr Professor Frank Schneider, sehr geehrte Damen und Herren, sehr geehrte Kolleginnen und Kollegen,

ich bin Sohn eines Neuropsychiaters, der gezwungen war, 1933 infolge der Nazi-Rassengesetze, plötzlich eine erfolgreiche medizinische Karriere in Deutschland aufgeben zu müssen. Ich war voller Erwartung, um vor diesem Plenum, vor Ihnen zu sprechen. Die Gedenkveranstaltung, an der Sie alle heute teilnehmen, ist ein wichtiger Meilenstein in der Aufarbeitung der Geschichte der deutschen Psychiatrie.

Leider kann ich, der ich selbst Psychiater bin, aus gesundheitlichen Gründen nicht persönlich an dem Kongress teilnehmen, und bin gezwungen, Ihnen meine Worte per Video zu übersenden. Diese Ansprache ist dem Andenken an meinen Vater, Dr. Kurt Blumenthal-Bental, und all denjenigen Psychiatern gewidmet, die ab 1933 gezwungen waren, plötzlich und unvermittelt, eine erfolgreiche medizinische Karriere und ein Leben in Deutschland aufzugeben, um in Palästina unter schwersten Bedingungen eine neue Laufbahn zu beginnen und ein neues Leben aufzubauen. Über 40 Psychiater, viele von ihnen in Deutschland in leitenden Posten tätig, wanderten damals nach Palästina/Israel aus.

Mein Vater Dr. Kurt Blumenthal, der seinen Namen in Israel 1949 zu Bental hebräisierte, wurde 1893 in Berlin geboren. Im Geiste der jüdischen Assimilation, des Liberalismus und der Aufklärung, die seit Anfang des 19. Jahrhunderts in Europa herrschten, wurde er erzogen und erhielt eine klassische deutsche Bildung mit Griechisch, Latein und Französisch sowie gründlichen Kenntnissen der deutschen und europäischen Literatur und Poesie. 1912 begann er sein Medizinstudium in Berlin, das er unterbrach, um als Medizinaloffizier im ersten Weltkrieg zu dienen.

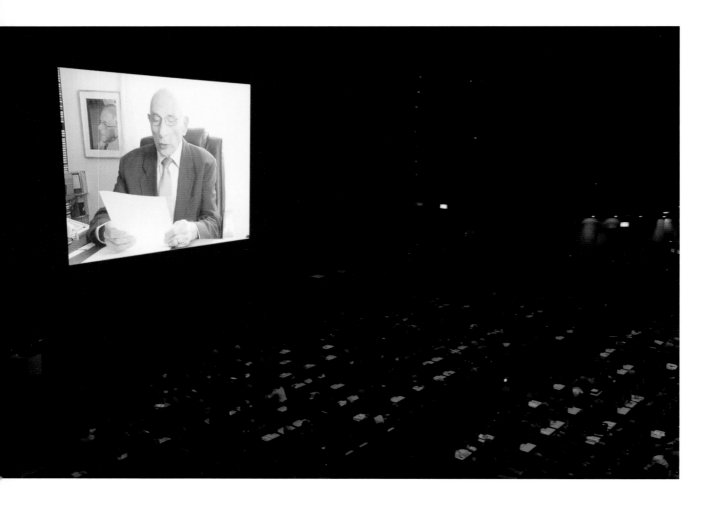

When the war ended he concluded his medical studies at the University of Rostock, where he received his doctoral degree in 1920. The title of his dissertation was: "Psychoses in hydrocephalus, meningitis serosa, cerebral edema and pseudotumor". He completed his professional training under Prof. Kleist at the psychiatric clinic in Rostock- Gelsheim and worked there until early 1923. He then moved to Dessau with his wife and young daughter, started his own neuropsychiatric practice, and held a position as a consultant at the psychiatric clinic of the local deaconess home.

My parents came out of the hardship that followed World War I as enlightened Germans who wanted to help build a just and democratic society. We three children were raised in the spirit of assimilation, firmly believing in peace and the good in people, not even being aware that we were Jews. Yet the outbreaks of anti-Semitism in Dessau in the early 1930s, as the Nazi movement gained momentum, brought about a radical shift in my parents' world view. The ideals and hopes which they had believed in fell apart.

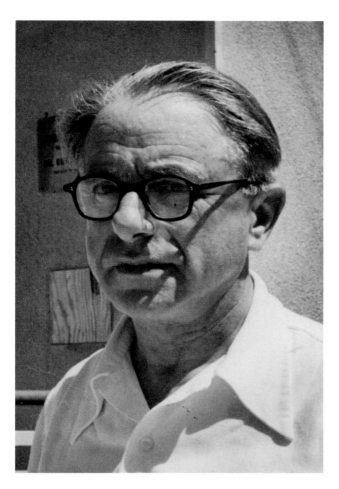

Dr. Kurt Blumenthal-Bental

Nach Ende des Krieges beendete er sein Medizinstudium an der Medizinischen Fakultät der Universität Rostock und erhielt dort 1920 den Doktortitel verliehen. Seine Arbeit hatte den Titel: „Psychosen bei Hydrocephalus, Meningitis serosa, Hirnschwellung und Pseudotumor". Seine Fachausbildung absolvierte er an der Nervenklinik Rostock-Gelsheim unter der Leitung von Prof. Dr. Kleist, wo er bis Anfang 1923 arbeitete. Danach zog die junge Familie – Frau und Tochter – nach Dessau, wo er eine Neuropsychiatrische Praxis gründete und als Konsiliarius an der Psychiatrischen Klinik des Diakonissenheimes amtierte.

Nach der schweren Nachkriegszeit fühlten sich meine Eltern als aufgeklärte Deutsche, die beim Aufbau einer demokratischen und gerechten Gesellschaft mitwirken wollten. Wir drei Kinder wurden im Geiste der Assimilation, im Glauben an den Frieden und an das Gute im Menschen erzogen, nicht bewusst, dass wir Juden waren. Die Weltanschauung unserer Eltern hat sich jedoch, angesichts der antisemitischen Ausbrüche in Dessau zu Beginn der dreißiger Jahre, als die Nazibewegung stärker wurde, grundsätzlich verändert. Die Ideale und Hoffnungen an die unsere Eltern geglaubt hatten, brachen zusammen.

I remember my teacher asking all of us pupils to bring a donation in order to buy a portrait of Hitler and hang it on the classroom wall. Being the only Jew in the class, my parents told me not to donate any money, thus I was despised and mocked by the other children as a Jew. My mother tried to explain to me, an eight-year old boy, what that notion, "Jew", meant. From there on, I stopped going to that school and was transferred to the Jewish school in the Klopstockstraße in Berlin.

One of my most shocking memories is, how on the first of April 1933, when I was a boy of eight years, I stood together with my sister and parents at the window of my father's practice at Antoinettenstraße 24 in Dessau, seeing the S.A. men standing in front of the house entrance with large signs that read:

GERMANS! DEFEND YOURSELVES!
DON'T GO TO JEWISH DOCTORS!

That was the decisive moment that prompted my parents to make their resolution that would change the rest of our lives. They decided: "In a country that does not want us, we will not stay."

Thus, the career of a successful young psychiatrist in Dessau terminated at that moment. My parents began to look for a country where they could take refuge to, and ultimately they decided on Palestine/Israel. They went ahead of us children and arrived in Haifa by late July 1933, where they tried to gain ground under extremely challenging conditions. They had to make a living and build up a new psychiatric practice from scratch in a country where they did not know the culture or the language and where living conditions were very difficult. We children arrived later and had to change our names. My name changed from Werni to Ephraim, my elder sister's name changed from Evi to Chawa, and my little brother Klausi became Benjamin.

Our parents had a very hard time adjusting to their new life, though we were not aware of it at the time. I had trouble with the language because of course they only spoke Hebrew at my school. A good illustration of our father's ability to courageously and resolutely look towards the future without regretting the past is the quote from Herrmann Hesse which he wrote on the first of July 1933, shortly before he left Germany, in my sister's friendship book:

"Children, do not hang your heads like that! Do not make old Zarathustra laugh! Is it a misfortune that you have been born into fresh, tempestuous, thunderous times? Is that not rather your good fortune?" *(Hermann Hesse: Zarathustras Wiederkehr, 1919)*

So kam es, dass der Klassenlehrer in meiner Schule alle Schüler um eine Geldspende bat, um ein Hitlerbild zu kaufen und in der Klasse aufzuhängen. Als ich als einziger Jude und auf meiner Eltern Anweisung hin keine Geldspende abgab, wurde ich von den Kindern der Klasse als Jude verpönt und verspottet. Meine Mutter versuchte mir, dem achtjährigem Jungen, zu erklären, was der Begriff Jude bedeutet. Von da an ging ich nicht mehr in diese Schule, sondern wurde in die jüdische Schule in der Klopstockstraße in Berlin umgeschult.

Eine meiner erschütterndsten Erinnerungen ist, wie ich am ersten April 1933 als achtjähriger Knabe gemeinsam mit meiner Schwester und unseren Eltern am Fenster der Praxis meines Vaters in der Antoinettenstraße 24 in Dessau stand und sah, wie auf der Straße vor dem Hauseingang SA-Männer mit großen Schildern standen, auf denen geschrieben war:

DEUTSCHE! WEHRT EUCH!
GEHT NICHT ZU JÜDISCHEN ÄRZTEN!

Dieser Moment gab den Ausschlag, in dem meine Eltern ihren Beschluss fassten, der fortan unser Leben prägen sollte: *„In einem Land, wo wir nicht gewollt sind, bleiben wir nicht."*

Die Laufbahn eines erfolgreichen jungen Psychiaters in Dessau, wurde in diesem Moment beendet. Auf der Suche nach einem Land, in dem sie Zuflucht finden könnten, fiel die endgültige Wahl unserer Eltern auf Palästina/Israel. Gemäß ihrem Beschluss landeten sie schon Ende Juli 1933 erst einmal allein in Haifa/Palästina, um dort, unter äußerst schwierigen Bedingungen zu versuchen, Fuß zu fassen, eine neue Existenz zu erschaffen und aufs Neue eine psychiatrische Praxis aufzubauen – in einem Land, dessen Sprache sie nicht kannten, dessen Lebensbedingungen schwierig und ihnen völlig fremd waren. Wir Kinder, die wir nachkamen, erhielten neue Namen: Ich wurde von Werni auf Ephraim umbenannt, meine ältere Schwester von Evi auf Chawa und mein jüngerer Bruder von Klausi auf Benjamin.

Die Umstellung war für unsere Eltern äußerst schwierig, aber wir Kinder waren dessen nicht so bewusst. Ich hatte Sprachschwierigkeiten, auf der Schule wurde ja nur Hebräisch gesprochen. Die Fähigkeit unseres Vaters, mit Mut und starken Willen in die Zukunft zu schauen, ohne das Vergangene zu bedauern, brachte er kurz vor seiner Abreise am ersten Juli 1933 mit einer Eintragung von Worten Friedrich Nietzsches im Poesiealbum meiner Schwester zum Ausdruck:

„Kinder, lasset die Köpfe nicht so herabhängen! Machet den alten Zarathustra nicht lachen! Ist es denn ein Unglück, dass ihr in frische, stürmische, brausende Zeiten hinein geboren seid? Ist denn das nicht euer Glück?" (Hermann Hesse: Zarathustras Wiederkehr, 1919)

Thus, slowly and with immense difficulties, my parents succeeded in laying the foundations for a new psychiatric hospital in Haifa. My father's persistence and determination, but also his doubts, often came to light in his diary, as the following entry from January 24, 1934 shows:

"I now have eight inpatients. Fewer patients came to the surgery in December, but January will be better. Unfortunately, we aren't getting a good night's rest because of course we can't afford a night nurse."

On February 6, 1934 he wrote:
"The practice was good in January, about 20 pounds. The house was also well occupied, which has enabled us to balance our budget. But Erna and I don't trust the lull. The house has not been fully utilized for three days now, and it is costing us more money than it generates, as we now have larger staff – one nurse and three auxiliary personnel."
(The nurse, Edith Katz, was a licensed nurse who had trained and worked at the Jewish hospital in Kassel. She became the head nurse at my father's clinic and stayed there until she retired in 1963.)

And on 8 April 1934:
"With eight patients, the house is well occupied. However, it is not enough to support us. The surgery hours have not developed any further. Each day with no new patients is agonizing."

Without any clear intentions or planning ahead, over time the tiny hospital grew into what was for those days a large, modern psychiatric clinic with 50 beds, and in 1937 it moved into a newly constructed, more suitable building on Mount Carmel in Haifa. It was known as the only centrally located psychiatric clinic in the entire northern part of the country. My father was the hospital's medical director, and five physicians worked there with him, as did care personnel and assistants. My mother was in charge of the business side.

Our family lived in the hospital building. This enabled me to begin gaining psychiatric experience while still young, since my father talked about his work during family meals.

Under my father's leadership, the clinic offered all of the newest treatments of those days, which are described in the medical literature of that time. The following deserve special mention:
1. Malaria treatment for progressive paralysis (which still existed in those days)
2. Insulin shock therapy (introduced at the clinic in 1937 by Dr. Rudi Meier, whom Dr. Blumenthal invited from Switzerland to work at the clinic)
3. Cardiazol shock treatment
4. Electroconvulsive treatment (using a machine that my father had requested to be especially built by an electrical engineer to specifications published in the medical literature by Ugo Cerletti and Lucio Bini in 1940)
5. Largactil treatment for acute psychoses (from 1952)
6. Leucotomies (performed according to the indications mentioned in the medical literature at that time)

Und so, langsam und unter großen Schwierigkeiten, gelang es meinen Eltern, in Haifa das Fundament für eine zukünftige psychiatrische Klinik zu legen. Meines Vaters Standhaftigkeit, seine Ausdauer und auch seine Zweifel, kamen in seinem Tagebuch oft zum Ausdruck, wie z. B. in der folgenden Eintragung vom 24. Januar 1934:

„Ich habe im Hause jetzt 8 Patienten. Die Sprechstunde war im Dezember ruhiger, aber der Januar wird schon besser. Leider haben wir keine richtige Nachtruhe, da wir uns natürlich keine Nachtschwester leisten können."

Am 6. Februar 1934 schreibt er:
„Die Praxis im Januar war gut, ca. 20 Pfund. Auch das Haus war gut belegt, sodass wir unseren Etat schon balanciert haben. Aber Erna und ich trauen dem Frieden nicht. Seit drei Tagen ist das Haus unterbelegt und kostet mehr als es bringt, denn wir haben jetzt einen ziemlich großen Apparat: eine Schwester und drei Mann Personal."
(Die Schwester war Edith Katz, diplomierte Krankenschwester, ehemals am jüdischen Krankenhaus in Kassel, die in der Klinik später als Oberschwester bis zu ihrer Pensionierung 1963 arbeitete.)

Und am 8. April 1934:
„Das Haus ist gut belegt: 8 Patienten. Aber das trägt unsere Existenz noch nicht. Die Sprechstundenpraxis hat sich nicht weiter entwickelt. Jeder Tag ohne Patientenzugang ist zermürbend."

Ohne klare Absichten oder Vorplanung am Anfang, entwickelte sich im Laufe der Zeit das kleine Krankenhaus in eine, für damalige Verhältnisse, große und moderne psychiatrische Klinik mit 50 Betten, die ab 1937 in ein neu gebautes, passenderes Gebäude auf dem Karmel in Haifa umzog. Das Haus war nun als einzige zentrale psychiatrische Klinik des ganzen Nordens anerkannt. Vater war der medizinische Leiter der Klinik, mit ihm arbeiteten fünf Ärzte sowie Pflegepersonal und Hilfskräfte. Mutter war die wirtschaftliche Leiterin.

Die Familie wohnte im Haus, so dass ich von Jugend her meine ersten psychiatrischen Erfahrungen bei den gemeinsamen Familienmahlzeiten mit Vater sammelte. Unter der Leitung meines Vaters wurden in der Klinik alle damals modernen Behandlungen eingeführt, so wie sie in der damaligen medizinischen Literatur beschrieben waren. Besonders erwähnt seien:
1. Malariabehandlung für Progressive Paralyse (damals noch vorkommend),
2. Insulinschocktherapie (eingeführt 1937 in der Klinik von Dr. Rudi Meier, den Dr. Blumenthal aus der Schweiz aufforderte, in der Klinik zu arbeiten),
3. Cardiazolschockbehandlung,
4. Elektrokrampfbehandlung (mit selbst gebautem Apparat auf Bestellung meines Vaters bei einem Elektroingenieur, gemäß den Angaben von Ugo Cerletti und Lucio Bini von 1940, die damals in der medizinischen Literatur veröffentlicht wurden),
5. Largactilbehandlung für akute Psychosen (ab 1952),
6. Leukotomien (empfohlen gemäß dem damaligen Stand der Literatur).

I would like to tell two anecdotes about the homemade electroconvulsive machine: To check that the machine was working properly, a cat was tied on a board on top of my father's desk, and the electrodes attached to its head. When the current was turned on, the cat received a shock and jumped out of the second-floor window, healthy and happy. With that the machine was pronounced suitable for use on humans and put it into regular operation.

This very machine played a role in the war declaration of Lebanon on Germany in early 1945. The Lebanon´s president was a patient of my father's and suffered from severe attacks of depression, which only responded to electroconvulsive treatment. The French government, which had the mandate over Lebanon, wanted Lebanon to declare war on Germany so it could become a member of the UN. Such a war declaration had to be signed by the president, but he was severely depressed and had little interest in anything. My father received an urgent call to go to Lebanon and give the statesman electroconvulsive treatment. After three treatments the president recovered and signed the war declaration. To show his thanks, he promised to grant any wish my father would make. In May 1946 my father heard that his dear Aunt Martha had returned to Berlin from the Theresienstadt concentration camp. Since there was no way of getting an immigration visa for Palestine my father asked the Lebanese president to give her an immigration visa to Lebanon. The president kept his promise and Aunt Martha got the visa. After a series of detours, she arrived in Haifa where she lived many happy years with the family.

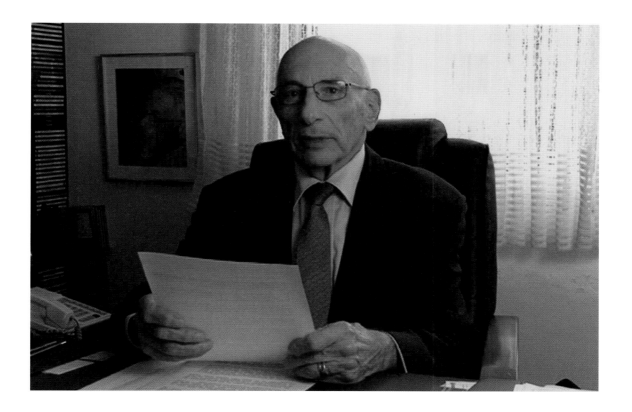

Zur Geschichte des selbstgebauten Elektrokrampfapparats möchte ich zwei Anekdoten erzählen: Um die Verlässlichkeit des Apparats zu prüfen, wurde eine Katze auf einem Brett auf dem Sprechstundenschreibtisch meines Vaters fixiert und die Elektroden an den Kopf angelegt. Der Strom wurde eingeschaltet, die Katze bekam einen Schock und sprang danach sofort durchs Fenster aus dem 2. Stock, gesund und munter. Damit war der Apparat als gebrauchsfähig für Menschen erklärt und wurde eingesetzt.

Dieser Apparat hat auch dazu beigetragen, dass der Libanon Anfang 1945 Deutschland den Krieg erklärt hat. Der damalige Präsident des Libanons war Patient meines Vaters und litt an schweren Depressionen, die nur auf Elektrokrampfbehandlung reagierten. Die französische Regierung, die das Mandat über den Libanon hatte, wollte, dass der Libanon Deutschland den Krieg erkläre, um damit das Recht in der Mitgliedschaft der UNO zu erhalten. Solch eine Kriegserklärung musste der Präsident persönlich unterschreiben, aber er war schwerst depressiv und wollte von nichts etwas wissen. Mein Vater wurde also dringend in den Libanon gerufen, um eine Elektrokrampfbehandlung durchzuführen. Nach drei Behandlungen erholte sich der Präsident und unterzeichnete die Kriegserklärung. Zum Dank versprach er, meinem Vater jeglichen Wunsch zu erfüllen. Im Mai 1946 erfuhr mein Vater, dass seine geliebte Tante Martha vom KZ Theresienstadt nach Berlin zurückgekehrt sei. Da es keine Möglichkeit gab, ein Einwanderungsvisum nach Palästina zu erhalten, bat nun mein Vater den Libanesischen Präsidenten um ein Einreisevisum für Tante Martha in den Libanon. Der Präsident hielt sein Versprechen und Tante Martha bekam das Visum. Sie kam auf Umwegen nach Haifa, wo sie noch viele glückliche Jahre im Kreise der Familie lebte.

My father managed the hospital until 1964 when the staff took it over and turned it into a cooperative. He still worked at the hospital as psychiatric consultant until 1973.

My father belonged to those neuropsychiatrists who were a common species at that time. Since I was the son of a psychiatrist and had grown up in a psychiatric clinic, it was obvious that I became a psychiatrist myself. I began my medical studies at the University of Bern and concluded them at the Hebrew University in Jerusalem, where I received my doctoral degree in medicine in 1954. I completed my professional training in neurology and psychiatry at the Department of Neurology at Hadassah University Hospital in Jerusalem. As a professor at the Medical School of the Technion in Haifa, I headed the neurology department at Rambam Hospital until 1991.

I am one of the few remaining neuropsychiatrists today, for which I have to thank my dear departed father. Our parents' "expulsion" from Germany helped give them the will and perseverance to found and run an outstanding, modern psychiatric clinic in Israel.

On a personal level, the sad turn of events in Germany led my parents, my siblings and me to find our way back to Judaism.

The generation of immigrated psychiatrists played an important and venerable role in the development of modern psychiatry in Israel. They learned to adapt to the special circumstances of the country despite enormous challenges at the outset. Because of them, a progressive psychiatry found its way to Israel, and they are the main reason it is taught and practiced nowadays.

May this event and my modest contribution to it be a worthy tribute to all the psychiatrists who were forced to leave Germany in the face of Nazi persecution. Modern Israeli psychiatry is what it is today in large part because of them.

Vater leitete die Klinik bis 1964, bis sie dann die Angestellten als Kooperative übernahmen. Bis 1973 arbeitete er noch als psychiatrischer Berater an der Klinik weiter.

Mein Vater gehörte zu der Klasse der Neuropsychiater, wie sie in der damaligen Zeit gang und gäbe waren. Da ich in einer psychiatrischen Klinik aufgewachsen bin, war es selbstverständlich, dass ich in die Fußtapfen meines Vaters trat. Ich begann mein Medizinstudium an der Medizinischen Fakultät Bern und beendete es an der Hebräischen Universität in Jerusalem, wo ich 1954 den Doktortitel der Medizin erhielt. An der Neurologischen Abteilung des Hadassah Universitätskrankenhauses Jerusalem absolvierte ich meine Fachausbildung in Neurologie und Psychiatrie. Als Professor an der Medizinischen Fakultät des Technions in Haifa leitete ich die Neurologische Abteilung des Rambamkrankenhauses bis 1991.

So gehöre ich heute noch zu den wenigen Neuropsychiatern. Dies habe ich hauptsächlich meinem seligen Vater zu verdanken. Die „Vertreibung" aus Deutschland hat dazu beigetragen dass unsere Eltern mit gutem Willen und viel Ausdauer eine hervorragende moderne Psychiatrische Klinik in Israel gründeten und leiteten.

Persönlich haben meine Eltern und wir Kinder, als Folge der traurigen Geschehnisse, unseren Rückweg zum Judentum gefunden.

Die Generation der emigrierten Psychiatern, die einen wichtigen und ehrenvollen Anteil an der Entwicklung der modernen Psychiatrie in Israel hat, hat es trotz enormer Anfangsschwierigkeiten verstanden, sich an die besonderen Umstände des Landes anzupassen. Ihnen ist zu verdanken, dass eine fortgeschrittene Psychiatrie im Lande eingeführt wurde und noch heute gelehrt und praktiziert wird.

Möge diese Veranstaltung und mein kleiner Beitrag dazu eine ehrenvolle Erinnerung an all die Psychiater sein, die aufgrund der Naziverfolgungen gezwungen waren, Deutschland zu verlassen. Sie haben einen großen Anteil am Aufbau einer modernen Psychiatrie in Israel.

Speech by Sigrid Falkenstein, Berlin, Relative of a victim

Ladies and gentlemen!

Today's commemorative event is particularly poignant for me, given the fatal link between my own family's history and the history of German psychiatry in the last century. As in many of the victims' families, my family repressed their memories of events and never spoke about the forced sterilisation and "euthanasia" that took place. You could say that this mirrors the collective process of denial in German society.

It was and is incomprehensible: the planned, organised mass murder of hundreds of thousands of sick and disabled people, perpetrated by those who were supposed to protect them, heal them and care for them. Why have we been silent on this issue for so long? How could we shy away from our responsibility?

Professor Schneider, as President of the German Association for Psychiatry and Psychotherapy (DGPPN) you are the first to officially acknowledge the perpetrators' guilt. You have expressed shame and sorrow, and asked the victims and their families for forgiveness for the suffering and injustice they were exposed to in the name of German psychiatry. I don't think it is going too far to describe this as a historical milestone, and I thank you for this.

The victims were not an anonymous mass – they were individuals, who were excluded, humiliated and finally murdered. Like my Aunt Anna, each one had a name and face – yet for decades these were wiped from memory.

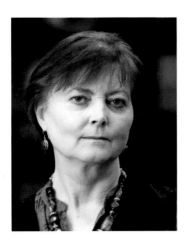

❯ Rede von Sigrid Falkenstein, Berlin, Angehörige eines Opfers

Sehr geehrte Damen und Herren,

die heutige Gedenkveranstaltung hat eine ganz besondere Bedeutung für mich, denn meine Familiengeschichte ist auf unheilvolle Weise mit der Geschichte der deutschen Psychiatrie im letzten Jahrhundert verbunden. Wie in vielen betroffenen Familien wurden Zwangssterilisation und „Euthanasie" auch in meiner Familie verschwiegen und verdrängt. Man kann wohl sagen, dass dies Spiegel eines kollektiven Verdrängungsprozesses der deutschen Gesellschaft insgesamt war.

Es ist und bleibt unfassbar: hunderttausendfacher, geplanter, organisierter Massenmord an kranken und behinderten Menschen, ausgeführt von denjenigen, die sie schützen, heilen und pflegen sollten. Wie konnte man das so lange verschweigen? Wie konnte man sich aus der Verantwortung dafür stehlen?

Sehr geehrter Herr Prof. Schneider, Sie haben vorhin als Präsident der Deutschen Gesellschaft für Psychiatrie, Psychotherapie und Nervenheilkunde (DGPPN) erstmals offiziell die Verantwortung der Täter benannt. Sie haben Scham und Trauer ausgedrückt und die Opfer sowie ihre Familien um Verzeihung gebeten für das Leid und das Unrecht, das ihnen im Namen der deutschen Psychiatrie angetan wurde. Vielleicht ist es nicht zu hoch gegriffen, dies als historischen Meilenstein zu bezeichnen! Ich danke Ihnen!

Die Opfer waren keine anonyme Masse, es waren einzelne Menschen, die ausgegrenzt, gedemütigt und am Ende vernichtet wurden. Sie alle hatten – wie meine Tante Anna – Namen und Gesicht, doch die Erinnerung an sie war jahrzehntelang ausgelöscht.

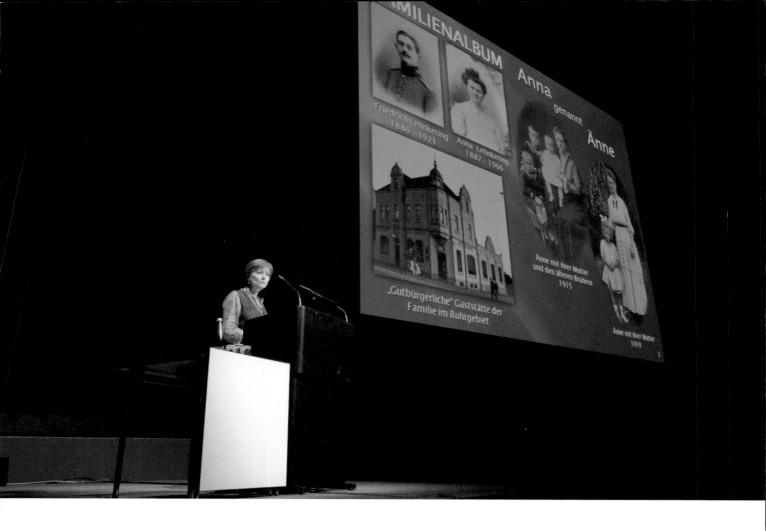

It is only recently that my aunt reentered my family's collective memory. Until 2003 I had only seen her in a few family photos and knew little about her. My grandparents, Friedrich and Anna Lehnkering, were middle-class restaurateurs in the Ruhr area. They had four children. Anna, who was sometimes called Änne, was their only daughter. My grandfather died in 1921, just one year after my father was born. Anna was six years old at the time. I was told that she, too, died young.

I was therefore shocked when in 2003, I stumbled across Anna's name on an online list of the victims of the Nazis' "euthanasia" programme. The research I then conducted with the help of Anna's medical records from the Federal Archives in Berlin revealed a whole new version of her life story. In 1935, she underwent forced sterilisation under the Law for the Prevention of Hereditarily Diseased Offspring. She had been diagnosed "congenitally feebleminded". From 1936 to 1940, Anna was a patient at the Bedburg-Hau mental hospital.

Her medical records include numerous entries – sometimes in unspeakable language – that document her psychological and physical decline. On the day she was admitted, Anna was described as calm and good-natured. To substantiate claims of her "congenital stupidity", she underwent an "intelligence test" that included strange questions like: "What is the difference between a child and a dwarf?" To this, her heart-warming answer was: "Children go to school and play. Dwarves wear pointy hats."

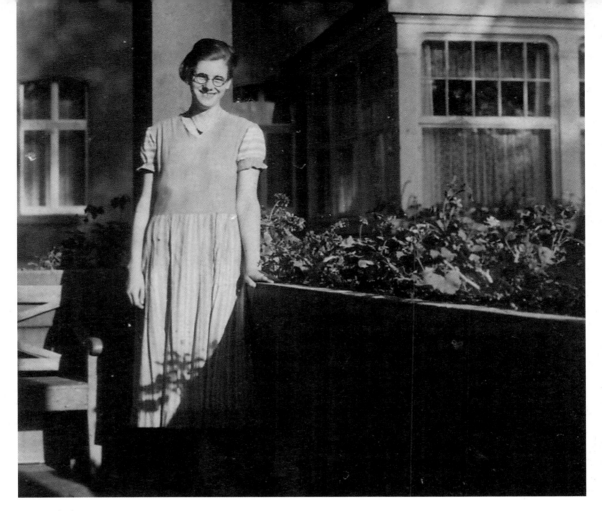

Anna Lehnkering

Meine Tante hat erst seit wenigen Jahren einen Platz im Familiengedächtnis. Bis 2003 kannte ich nur einige Familienfotos und wusste kaum etwas über sie. Meine Großeltern Friedrich und Anna Lehnkering stammten beide aus bürgerlichem Milieu im Ruhrgebiet und betrieben dort eine Gaststätte. Sie hatten vier Kinder. Anna, die auch Änne genannt wurde, war die einzige Tochter. Mein Großvater starb bereits 1921, nur ein Jahr nach der Geburt meines Vaters. Anna war damals sechs Jahre alt. Man hatte mir erzählt, dass sie ebenfalls jung gestorben wäre.

So war es ein Schock, als ich 2003 per Zufall im Internet auf Annas Namen stieß. Er stand auf einer Liste von Opfern der nationalsozialistischen „Euthanasie"-Aktion. Meine nun folgende Spurensuche mithilfe von Annas Patientenakte aus dem Berliner Bundesarchiv ergab ein völlig neues Bild ihrer Lebensgeschichte. 1935 wurde sie auf Grundlage des „Gesetzes zur Verhütung erbkranken Nachwuchses" zwangssterilisiert. Die Diagnose ihrer Krankheit lautete „angeborener Schwachsinn". Von 1936 bis 1940 war Anna Patientin in der Heil- und Pflegeanstalt Bedburg-Hau.

In Annas Krankenblatt gibt es viele – teils in einer unsäglichen Sprache verfasste – Eintragungen, die ihren seelischen und körperlichen Verfall dokumentieren. Am Tag ihrer Aufnahme ist sie ruhig und verträglich. Zur Untermauerung ihrer „erblichen Dummheit" muss Anna sich einer „Intelligenzprüfung" unterziehen. So stellt man ihr beispielsweise die merkwürdige Frage nach dem Unterschied zwischen einem Kind und einem Zwerg. Ihre rührende Antwort lautet: „Kinder gehen in die Schule und spielen. Zwerge haben Zipfelmützen auf."

The records go on to say that Anna cried a lot during her first weeks at Bedburg-Hau and wanted to go home. Who could blame her? She is then described as an increasingly difficult patient. Notes about her include that she "refuses to work", that she "encourages disobedience in other patients", that she is "unhygienic", and that she "has to be disciplined." Just how treacherous language can be is shown in remarks like "she blubbers; she is foolish". The worst of all these callous comments is the note that describes Anna as "a burden". At the end of her time at the mental hospital, she bore clear signs of malnourishment and of tuberculosis.

As the records did not reveal where or how Anna died, I targeted the administration at Bedburg-Hau. After a long silence, I received a brief message informing me that on 6 March 1940 my aunt was transferred to Grafeneck, where she passed away on 23 April 1940.

I now know what really happened. Transferred, passed away – such harmless words! Not even the date of her death was correct! In a period of just four days in March 1940, Bedburg Hau's 1 600 plus patients were deported en masse so the facilities could be used as a military hospital. Along with 455 other patients, Anna was deported to Grafeneck, where she was murdered in a gas chamber disguised as a shower. And it was actually a physician who turned on the gas.

The "Aktion T4" programme in Grafeneck marked the beginning of the systematic, industrial mass murder that would culminate in the Holocaust.

Anna fulfilled her murderers' selection criteria perfectly. She was not only "incurably hereditarily diseased" according to Nazi ideology, but was considered "economically unusable" and therefore "human ballast", a "useless eater". With the simple bureaucratic act of marking a red plus sign on a form, some medical experts here in Berlin whom she had never met designated her "unworthy of life" and sent her to her death. Anna was just 24 years old.

Those are merely the facts – the harrowing images that lie beneath them elude our imaginations.

Somehow, my family knew nothing of this story. It seemed to me as if these terrible events had been completely erased from memory. My father can only remember fragments of his sister's life. These are mostly happy memories from his childhood and youth. He told me that Anna was very sweet and good-natured. She had learning difficulties and therefore went to a special school. Later she helped their mother out with the family business. However, there are "black holes" in my father's memory when it comes to the period from 1936 to 1940.

Weiterhin liest man im Krankenblatt, dass Anna in den ersten Wochen in Bedburg-Hau sehr viel weint, sie möchte nach Hause. Wer will es ihr verdenken? Dann wird sie als zunehmend schwierige Patientin beschrieben. Es heißt unter anderem: Sie „verweigert die Arbeit", sie „hetzt andere Kranke auf", sie ist „unsauber" und „muss zur Ordnung angehalten werden". Wie verräterisch Sprache sein kann, zeigen Vermerke wie „sie plärrt, sie ist läppisch". Der Gipfel solch menschenverachtender Bemerkungen ist die Notiz, dass Anna „lästig" sei. Am Ende ist sie schwer gezeichnet durch Mangelernährung und Tuberkulose.

Da aus der Krankenakte nicht hervorgeht, wo und wie Anna starb, ging meine Spurensuche in Bedburg-Hau weiter. Nach langem Schweigen bekam ich von dort die lapidare Auskunft, dass meine Tante am 6. März 1940 nach Grafeneck verlegt wurde, wo sie am 23. April 1940 verstarb.

Inzwischen hatte ich mich informiert. Verlegt, verstarb – welch beschönigenden Worte! Noch nicht einmal das Todesdatum stimmte! Im März 1940 kam es in Bedburg-Hau innerhalb von vier Tagen zu einer Massendeportation von mehr als 1 600 Patienten und Patientinnen, um Platz für ein Marinelazarett zu schaffen. Anna wurde zusammen mit 455 anderen Kranken nach Grafeneck deportiert, wo sie umgehend in einer als Duschraum getarnten Gaskammer ermordet wurde. Es war ein Arzt, der den Gashebel persönlich bediente.

In Grafeneck begann mit der „Aktion T4" die systematisch-industrielle Vernichtung von Menschen, die letztlich in den Holocaust mündete.

Anna erfüllte die Selektionskriterien ihrer Mörder perfekt. Sie galt nicht nur im Sinne der NS-Rassenideologie als „unheilbar erbkrank", sondern sie war auch „ökonomisch unbrauchbar" und damit eine „Ballastexistenz", eine „nutzlose Esserin". Mit einem bloßen bürokratischen Akt, einem roten Plus im Meldebogen, wurde sie von ärztlichen Gutachtern hier in Berlin, die sie noch nicht einmal kannten, als „lebensunwert" zur Vernichtung bestimmt. Anna wurde nur 24 Jahre alt.

Soweit die bloßen Fakten – die grauenvollen Bilder, die sich dahinter auftun, entziehen sich jeder Vorstellungskraft.

Von dieser Geschichte war nichts im Familiengedächtnis vorhanden. Es schien mir, als ob die schlimmen Geschehnisse geradezu ausgeblendet worden wären. Mein Vater erinnerte sich nur noch bruchstückhaft. Überwiegend schöne Erinnerungen an Kindheit und Jugend waren geblieben. Er erzählte mir, dass Anna eine sehr liebe und gutmütige Schwester war. Sie hatte Schwierigkeiten beim Lernen, darum ging sie zu einer Hilfsschule. Später half sie der Mutter im Geschäftshaushalt. In Bezug auf die Zeit zwischen 1936 und 1940 gab es „schwarze Löcher" im Gedächtnis.

Perhaps a photo can help explain. It shows my father as a boy of around 12 looking affectionately and protectively at his sister. Just a few years later – when he was 16 – Anna was separated from her family. He was a 19-year-old soldier, far away from home, when she was murdered. He couldn't help her; he couldn't protect her. I can only speculate that it is his feelings of guilt and shame that caused these "black holes" in his memory.

I found other explanations for these gaps and this incredible mass "forgetting" after I had delved into the history of Nazi eugenics and taken a look at my family's "genealogical chart".

The genealogical chart encompasses 24 people. It is mostly based on denunciations and hearsay, and is a mixture of truth and lies. Aside from Anna, three other relations were designated "hereditarily inferior". Among them was my grandfather who had died in the early Twenties – he had been an alcoholic and was therefore deemed "debauched". The descriptions of individual family members' character traits are ludicrous – it is hard to believe that such pseudoscientific nonsense was ever written by physicians.

No matter how true or untrue the entries about my family are, like any other family mine is and was a colourful mixture of individuals with different dispositions, skills and inclinations whose development has been influenced by various external forces. In any case, the theory of our family's "congenital stupidity" has no proven basis, as most of my grandparents' descendants have had an excellent school or university education – although this is by no means a sign of "congenital intelligence" either!

After WWII, Anna was never mentioned in the family. Perhaps this is because there were other problems to deal with in the post-war period, like where the next meal was coming from. Perhaps the family – like much of society – had come to believe in Nazi doctrine on hereditary health. Whatever the reasons, they tried hard to keep up the façade of a "respectable middle-class way of life", and the "hereditary inferiority" label certainly didn't fit in with that. My grandmother suffered from severe geriatric depression in later life, and it is likely that the repression of the traumatic experiences within her family played a major role in this.

My aunt's unimaginable suffering profoundly moved me. But I was also at a loss to comprehend my family's and society's silence on the issue. These experiences have motivated me in my research into the past.

Vielleicht trägt ein Foto zur Erklärung bei. Es zeigt, wie mein Vater als etwa 12-jähriger Junge liebevoll und beschützend auf seine Schwester blickt. Nur wenige Jahre später, er war 16, wurde Anna von der Familie getrennt. Er war 19-jähriger Soldat, weit weg von zu Hause, als sie ermordet wurde. Er konnte ihr nicht helfen, er konnte sie nicht beschützen. Ich kann nur spekulieren, dass auch Schuld- und Schamgefühle zu den „schwarzen Löchern" in seinem Gedächtnis geführt haben.

Weitere Erklärungen für dieses unglaubliche Nichtwissen und „Vergessen" fand ich, nachdem ich mich mit der Geschichte der NS-Rassenhygiene befasst hatte und Zusammenhänge mit der Sippentafel der Familie herstellte.

Die Sippentafel erfasst 24 Personen. Sie beruht größtenteils auf Denunziation und Hörensagen und ist eine Mischung aus Wahrheit und Lüge. Außer Anna werden noch drei andere Verwandte als „erblich minderwertig" diskriminiert. Dazu gehört auch mein bereits Anfang der 20er Jahre verstorbener Großvater, der alkoholkrank war und als „liederlich" abgewertet wird. Die Beschreibung der Charaktereigenschaften einzelner Familienmitglieder ist aberwitzig – nicht nachvollziehbar, dass solch ein pseudowissenschaftlich getarnter Unsinn von Ärzten unterzeichnet wurde.

Egal, wie wahr oder unwahr die Eintragungen sind, unsere Familie ist – wie jede Familie – eine bunte Mischung von Individuen mit verschiedenen Anlagen, Fähigkeiten und Neigungen, deren Entwicklungen von vielfältigen äußeren Einflüssen geprägt wurden. Auf jeden Fall lässt sich anhand unserer Familie die These „erblicher Dummheit" nicht beweisen, denn die meisten Nachkommen meiner Großeltern haben eine höhere Schulbildung oder einen Hochschulabschluss – was sicher im Umkehrschluss auch nicht als Zeichen „erblicher Intelligenz" zu deuten ist!

Nach dem 2. Weltkrieg war Anna kein Thema in der Familie. Vielleicht lag es daran, dass man in der schweren Nachkriegszeit andere, existenzielle Sorgen hatte. Vielleicht war die Familie – wie weite Teile der Gesellschaft – indoktriniert durch die „Lehre von der Erbgesundheit". Auf jeden Fall war sie bemüht, die Fassade einer „wohlanständigen Bürgerlichkeit" zu wahren. Dazu passte nicht der Makel „erblicher Minderwertigkeit". Meine Großmutter litt später an schweren Altersdepressionen. Es ist zu vermuten, dass das Verdrängen ihrer traumatischen familiären Erfahrungen eine große Rolle dabei spielte.

Das unvorstellbare Leid meiner Tante hat mich zutiefst berührt. Unfassbar fand ich aber auch das familiäre und gesellschaftliche Schweigen darüber. Diese Erfahrungen sind die Triebfeder für meine persönliche Erinnerungsarbeit.

Anna has now been commemorated in several ways:

- I set up a website in her honour in 2004.[1]
- Through it, the artist Ulrike Oeter found out about Anna and created the commemorative installation Aenne's letzte Reise [Aenne's last journey]. The clinic in Bedburg-Hau bought the artwork and since 2009 Anna's face has thus featured in the clinic's museum as a representative of all the other victims.
- As a typical example of how people with disabilities were treated under National Socialism, Anna's story is included in the school textbook Zeiten und Menschen [Times and people].
- Following the logic that "A person is only forgotten when his or her name is forgotten," a Stolperstein (literally "stumbling block") was laid for her in 2009. [Translator's note: A Stolperstein is a cobblestone-sized block laid outside the former house of a victim of the Nazi regime. They are inscribed with the victim's name and details.]

Today Anna has a firm place in our family's memory. I'm happy that my family were understanding about my research. My father in particular went through a painful – and hopefully liberating – process of remembering. On the day Anna's Stolperstein was laid, he publicly acknowledged his disabled sister for the first time. He died just a few weeks later. The words he directed at me – "Thank you for all that you have done for Änne" – meant a lot to me.

The change in public perception of Nazi medical crimes certainly owes much to the internet and the opportunities it opens up for communicating and sharing information. Since starting the website for Anna in 2004, I've had frequent messages from the relatives of other victims. There is a common thread running through all these letters: the issue of forced sterilisation and "euthanasia" has always been a family taboo, sometimes right up to the present day. Not infrequently, shame and the stigma of being related to someone with a psychological illness or who is mentally disabled play a role in this. However, more and more relatives are now publishing books, websites and other documentation to help them come to terms with their family's history and to give faces and names, and therefore some individuality and dignity, back to the victims.

For a long time and at all levels of society – in politics, administration, the judicial system, the Church and other institutions – any attempt to come to terms with the past met with resistance. This was also reflected in the media's scant interest in the subject, which has now slowly started to revive.

---

[1] http://www.sigrid-falkenstein.de/euthanasie/anna.htm

Für Anna gibt es inzwischen verschiedene Gedenkzeichen:

- 2004 habe ich eine Internet-Gedenkseite für sie gestaltet.[1]
- Die Künstlerin Ulrike Oeter wurde dadurch auf Anna aufmerksam und schuf die Installation der Erinnerung „Aennes letzte Reise". Das Kunstwerk wurde inzwischen von der Klinik in Bedburg-Hau erworben und zeigt Annas Gesicht seit 2009 stellvertretend für die anderen Opfer im Klinikmuseum.
- Annas Schicksal hat als exemplarisches Beispiel für den Umgang mit behinderten Menschen während des Nationalsozialismus Eingang in das Geschichtsbuch „Zeiten und Menschen" gefunden.
- 2009 wurde unter dem Motto „Ein Mensch ist erst vergessen, wenn sein Name vergessen ist" ein Stolperstein für sie verlegt.

Anna hat heute einen festen Platz im Familiengedächtnis. Ich bin froh, dass meine Spurensuche in der Familie weitestgehend auf Verständnis stieß. Vor allem mein Vater stellte sich einem schmerzhaften – hoffentlich auch für ihn „befreienden" – Erinnerungsprozess. Am Tag der Stolpersteinverlegung bekannte er sich erstmals öffentlich zu seiner behinderten Schwester. Er starb nur wenige Wochen später. Seine an mich gerichteten Worte: „Danke für alles, was du für Änne getan hast", bedeuten mir viel.

Der Wandel in der öffentlichen Wahrnehmung der NS-Medizinverbrechen hat sicher auch mit dem Internet und seinen vielfältigen Informationen und Kommunikationsmöglichkeiten zu tun. Seitdem ich 2004 die Internetseite für Anna veröffentlicht habe, bekomme ich immer wieder Zuschriften von anderen betroffenen Angehörigen. Es gibt eine Gemeinsamkeit: Das Thema Zwangssterilisation und „Euthanasie" wurde – und wird teilweise bis in die Gegenwart – in den Familien tabuisiert. Nicht selten spielen Scham und die Stigmatisierung als Angehörige von psychisch kranken und geistig behinderten Menschen eine Rolle. Aber mit Büchern, Internetseiten oder anderen Dokumentationen arbeiten immer mehr Angehörige ihre Familiengeschichten auf und geben den Opfern Gesicht und Namen und damit wenigstens einen Teil ihrer Persönlichkeit und Würde zurück.

Politik, Verwaltung, Justiz, Kirche, beteiligte Institutionen – auf allen gesellschaftlichen Ebenen hat man sich lange Zeit gegen das Aufarbeiten der Vergangenheit gesperrt. Das spiegelte sich auch in dem sehr geringen Interesse der Medien wider, das erst in letzter Zeit langsam zunimmt.

---

[1] http://www.sigrid-falkenstein.de/euthanasie/anna.htm

Tearing down this wall of silence required a new, impartial generation that was not tangled up in the events of the past. In the early Eighties young doctors started asking awkward questions about the past, and were often attacked for fouling their own nest. An event like today's is probably only possible because those young doctors are now in positions of power.

Now it is not just memorials in places where "euthanasia" crimes were committed that call these atrocities to mind. Recent years have also seen more historical research and greater efforts to encourage education on the subject.

However, remembrance work in our society is still largely driven by the tireless work of small local initiatives and concerned citizens. Among them are many people suffering from psychological illness and mental disabilities who know very well what it is to be socially excluded.

Almost 71 years after this systematic murder of sick and disabled people began, the issue has still not been properly addressed in the German culture of remembrance. When I say this I am thinking of the sorry state of the T4 memorial in Berlin, which still stands as a symbol for silence and "forgetting". Along with many others, I advocate the construction of a central, national memorial and documentation site in Tiergartenstrasse, the place where the "euthanasia" murders were planned and organised.

In a time of controversial debates on medicine and bioethics, such memorials are important – not only as places of remembrance, but also as information sites. History teaches us what happens in a society that views human beings as mere objects for medical opportunities and, finally only assesses them according to their usefulness.

I had the great honour of meeting sculptor and author Dorothea Buck. She, herself labelled "inferior" and forcibly sterilised, left me with the following words: "Terrible happenings that are not remembered can reoccur any time living conditions appreciably decline". In view of this, alarm bells should start ringing when – as recently – eugenic theories about socioeconomically valuable and less valuable life start to circulate in our country and when people start talking nonsense about the "congenital stupidity" of entire demographic groups.

Um die Mauern des Schweigens einzureißen, war sicher eine neue, unbefangenere Generation nötig, die nicht in die Geschehnisse verstrickt war. Dazu gehörten auch junge Ärzte, die etwa seit Beginn der 80er Jahre angefangen haben, unbequeme Fragen nach der Vergangenheit zu stellen und dafür nicht selten als „Nestbeschmutzer" beschimpft wurden. Dass eine Veranstaltung wie die heutige möglich ist, hat möglicherweise auch damit zu tun, dass jene jungen Ärzte heute in verantwortlichen Positionen sind.

Inzwischen widmet man sich nicht nur in den Gedenkstätten an den Orten der „Euthanasie"-Verbrechen den Aufgaben des Gedenkens und Mahnens. In den letzten Jahren kamen verstärkt historische Forschung und Bildungsarbeit hinzu.

Es bleibt jedoch festzuhalten, dass der Anstoß für diese gesellschaftliche Erinnerungsarbeit vor allem durch bürgerschaftliches Engagement gegeben wurde und das bleibende Verdienst kleiner, lokaler Initiativen und einzelner Menschen ist. Darunter sind nicht wenige, die heute von psychischen Krankheiten und Behinderung betroffen sind und nach wie vor erfahren, was gesellschaftliche Exklusion bedeutet.

Fast 71 Jahre nach Beginn der Krankenmorde gibt es leider immer noch Defizite in Bezug auf die deutsche Erinnerungskultur. Dabei denke ich auch an den unangemessenen Zustand des „T4"-Gedenkortes in Berlin, der ein Symbol für das Verschweigen und Vergessen ist. Zusammen mit vielen anderen Menschen setze ich mich für die Errichtung eines zentralen, nationalen Gedenk- und Dokumentationsortes am historischen Standort der Planung und Organisation der „Euthanasie"-Morde an der Tiergartenstraße ein.

In einer Zeit schwieriger medizin- und bioethischer Debatten ist ein solcher Ort wichtig – nicht nur als Ort des Gedenkens, sondern vor allem als Ort der Information. Die Geschichte lehrt uns doch, was mit einer Gesellschaft passieren kann, die Menschen zu bloßen Objekten medizinischer Möglichkeiten macht und letztendlich nur nach ihrem Nutzwert bemisst.

Ich hatte die große Ehre die Bildhauerin und Autorin Dorothea Buck kennenzulernen. Sie, die selbst als „minderwertig" abgestempelt und zwangssterilisiert wurde, hat mir folgenden Satz mit auf den Weg gegeben: „Was nicht erinnert wird, kann jederzeit wieder geschehen, wenn die äußeren Lebensumstände sich entscheidend verschlechtern." In diesem Zusammenhang müssten alle Alarmglocken schrillen, wenn – wie unlängst geschehen – eugenische Thesen über sozioökonomisch wertvolles und weniger wertvolles Leben in unserem Land kursieren, und über die „erbliche Dummheit" ganzer Bevölkerungsgruppen schwadroniert wird.

Ladies and gentlemen, we have a common responsibility to nip such developments in the bud and to challenge these inhuman views! We must learn from the past and use the memory of Anna and the other victims to help us shape an inclusive society built on solidarity, a society that values the individuality and diversity of all its members!

Prof. Schneider, today the DGPPN has made a very late but nevertheless very important step. You have paid tribute to the victims, and therefore given them and their families the respect and honour they were denied for so long. For that, and for your promise to put your weight behind efforts to promote the dignity and human rights of all people, I would like to thank you and all those present who take these commitments seriously.

Sehr geehrte Damen und Herren, es liegt in unserer gemeinsamen Verantwortung, den Anfängen zu wehren und solchen menschenverachtenden Einstellungen entschieden entgegenzutreten! Lassen Sie uns aus der Geschichte lernen und die Erinnerung an Anna und die anderen Opfer als Orientierungshilfe nutzen bei der Gestaltung einer solidarischen, inklusiven Gesellschaft, einer Gesellschaft, die niemanden ausgrenzt und Individualität und Vielfalt der Menschen wertschätzt!

Sehr geehrter Herr Prof. Schneider, mit dem heutigen Tag hat die DGPPN ein sehr spätes, aber darum nicht weniger wichtiges Zeichen gesetzt. Sie würdigt die Opfer und erweist ihnen und ihren Familien damit im Nachhinein Respekt und Ehre, die ihnen so lange verweigert wurden. Dafür und für das Versprechen, gemeinsam für die Achtung der Würde und Rechte aller Menschen zu arbeiten, danke ich Ihnen und allen Anwesenden, denen es mit diesem Bekenntnis ernst ist.

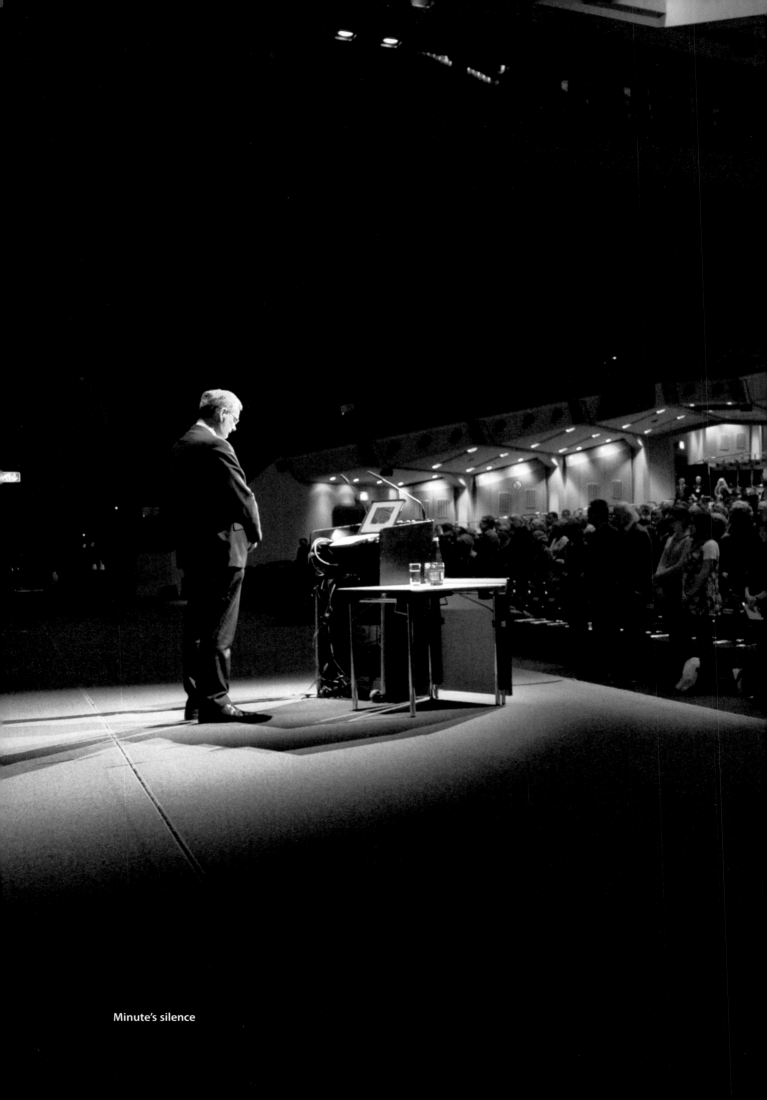

Minute's silence

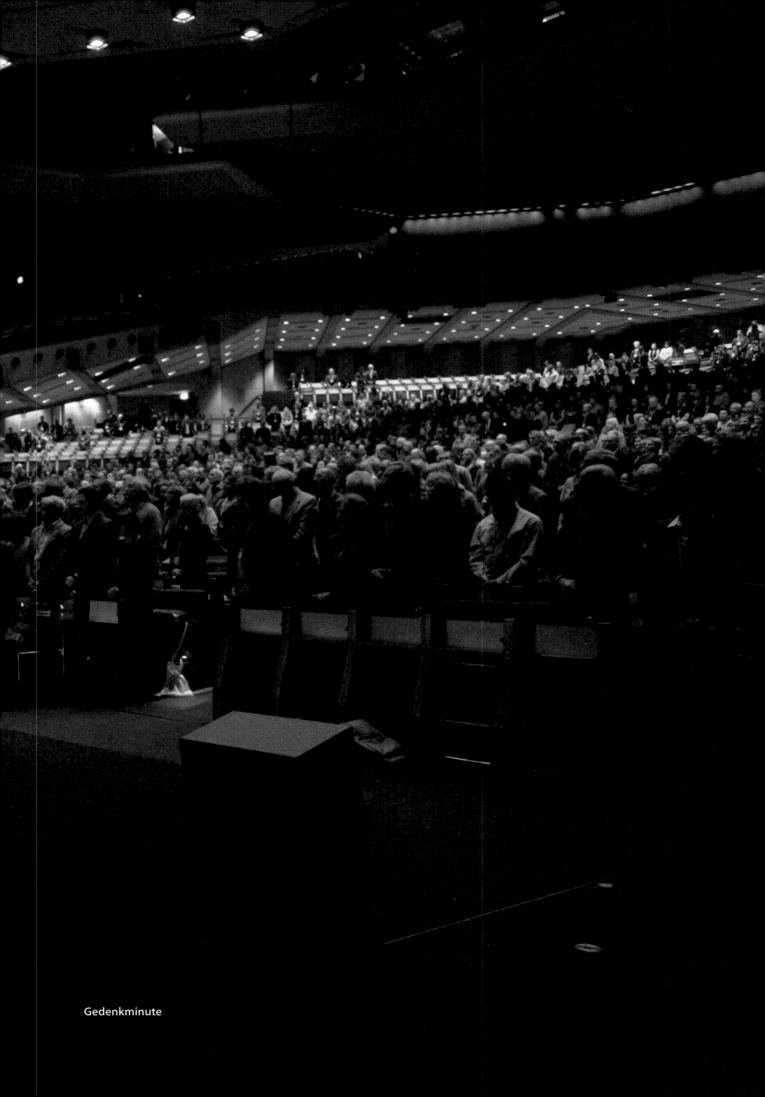

Gedenkminute

Psychiatry under National Socialism – Remembrance and Responsibility

Program of the Commemorative Event

Press conference
Psychiatry under National Socialism: Victims and Perpetrators
Prof. Dr. Dr. Frank Schneider, Aachen
President of the German Association for Psychiatry and Psychotherapy (DGPPN)
The Obligation of the DGPPN to Accept its Responsibility for the Crimes of the Past

Prof. Dr. Volker Roelcke, Gießen
Head of the "Commission to Investigate the History of the DGPPN"
The Current Status of Historical Research into the Role of Psychiatry under National Socialism

Prof. Dr. Michael von Cranach, Munich
Learning from the Past

Prof. Dr. Paul Weindling, Oxford
Member of the "Commission to Investigate the History of the DGPPN"
In the Shadow of Psychiatry: the Victims of Coercive Research under National Socialism

Ruth Fricke, Herford
Federal Organisation of (ex-) Users and Survivors of Psychiatry in Germany (BPE)
The Forgotten Victims

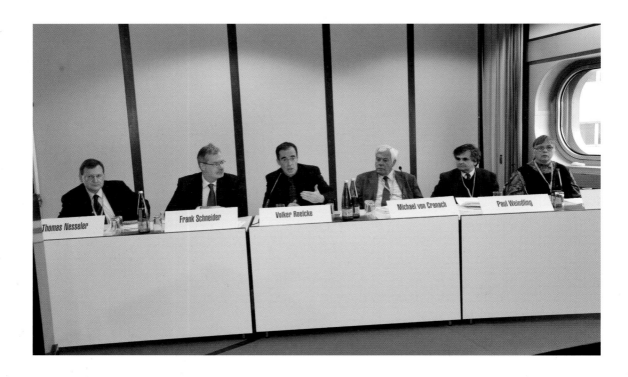

Psychiatrie im Nationalsozialismus – Erinnerung und Verantwortung

Ablauf des Gedenktags

Pressegespräch
Psychiatrie im Nationalsozialismus: Opfer und Täter
Prof. Dr. Dr. Frank Schneider, Aachen
Präsident der Deutschen Gesellschaft für Psychiatrie, Psychotherapie und Nervenheilkunde
(DGPPN)
Die Verpflichtung der DGPPN, sich der Vergangenheit zu stellen

Prof. Dr. Volker Roelcke, Gießen
Vorsitzender der „Kommission zur Aufarbeitung der Geschichte der DGPPN"
Der gegenwärtige Stand der historischen Forschung zur Rolle der Psychiatrie im Nationalsozialismus

Prof. Dr. Michael von Cranach, München
Von der Geschichte lernen

Prof. Dr. Paul Weindling, Oxford
Mitglied der „Kommission zur Aufarbeitung der Geschichte der DGPPN"
Im Schatten der Psychiatrie: Die Opfer von erzwungener Forschung im Nationalsozialismus

Ruth Fricke, Herford
Bundesverband Psychiatrie-Erfahrener e.V. (BPE)
Die vergessenen Opfer

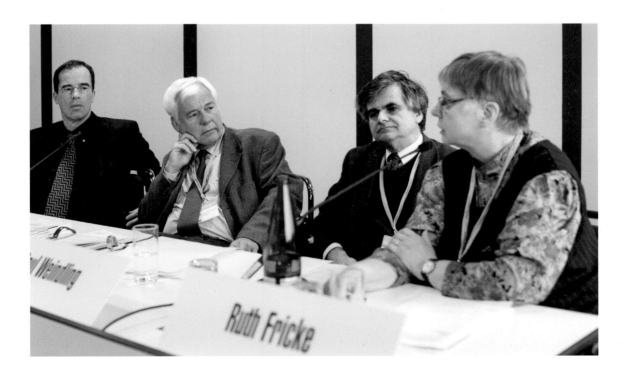

President's Symposium
Psychiatry under National Socialism
Chair: Prof. Dr. Dr. Frank Schneider (Aachen), Prof. Dr. Volker Roelcke (Gießen)

Prof. Dr. Volker Roelcke, Gießen University, Institute for the History of Medicine
Psychiatry under National Socialism – Historical Findings, Open Questions

Prof. Dr. Carola Sachse, University of Vienna, Department of Contemporary History
Dealing with the Past post-1945 in the Biomedical Sciences: the Example of the Max Planck Society

Prof. Dr. Hans-Walter Schmuhl, ZeitSprung/Kórima e.V. (Bielefeld)
Backing Each Other Up? The Society of German Neurologists and Psychiatrists and the "Gesundheitsführung" [Health Control] of National Socialism

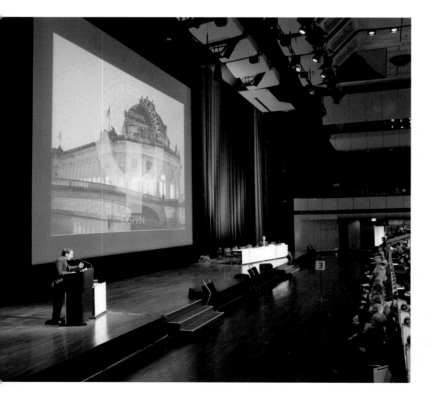
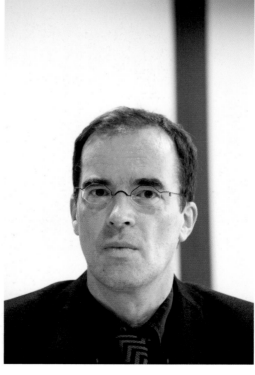

Prof. Dr. Volker Roelcke

Präsidentensymposium

Psychiatrie im Nationalsozialismus

Vorsitz: Prof. Dr. Dr. Frank Schneider (Aachen), Prof. Dr. Volker Roelcke (Gießen)

Prof. Dr. Volker Roelcke, Universität Gießen, Institut für Geschichte der Medizin
Psychiatrie im Nationalsozialismus – Historische Kenntnisse, offene Fragen

Prof. Dr. Carola Sachse, Universität Wien, Institut für Zeitgeschichte
Vergangenheitspolitik nach 1945 in den biomedizinischen Wissenschaften: Das Beispiel der Max-Planck-Gesellschaft

Prof. Dr. Hans-Walter Schmuhl, Agentur ZeitSprung/Kórima e.V. (Bielefeld)
Ressourcen füreinander? Die Gesellschaft Deutscher Neurologen und Psychiater und die national-sozialistische „Gesundheitsführung"

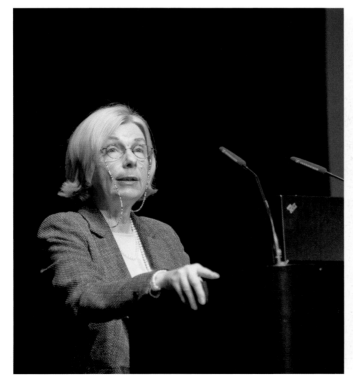
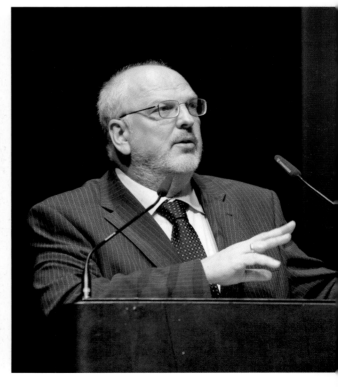

Prof. Dr. Carola Sachse   Prof. Dr. Hans-Walter Schmuhl

Commemorative Event

Psychiatry under National Socialism – Remembrance and Responsibility

Reading of documents relating to forced sterilisation and the killing of patients under National Socialism

Speakers: Peter Veit (Munich) and Simone Schatz (Irsee)

Selection and concept: Prof. Dr. Michael von Cranach (Eggenthal), PD Dr. Gerrit Hohendorf (Munich) and Dr. Maike Rotzoll (Heidelberg)

Speech by DGPPN President

Prof. Dr. Dr. Frank Schneider (Aachen)

Speeches by victim's representatives

Prof. Dr. Ephraim Bental (Haifa)

Sigrid Falkenstein (Berlin)

Minute's silence

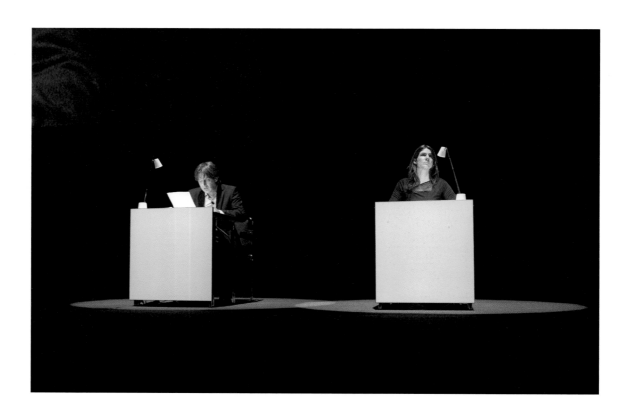

Gedenkveranstaltung

Psychiatrie im Nationalsozialismus – Erinnerung und Verantwortung

Dokumentenlesung zu Zwangssterilisation und Krankenmord im Nationalsozialismus

Sprecher: Peter Veit (München) und Simone Schatz (Irsee)

Auswahl der Dokumente und Konzept: Prof. Dr. Michael von Cranach (Eggenthal), Priv.-Doz. Dr. Gerrit Hohendorf (München) und Dr. Maike Rotzoll (Heidelberg)

Erklärung des Präsidenten der DGPPN

Prof. Dr. Dr. Frank Schneider (Aachen)

Erklärungen von Repräsentanten der Opfergruppen

Prof. Dr. Ephraim Bental (Haifa)

Sigrid Falkenstein (Berlin)

Gedenkminute

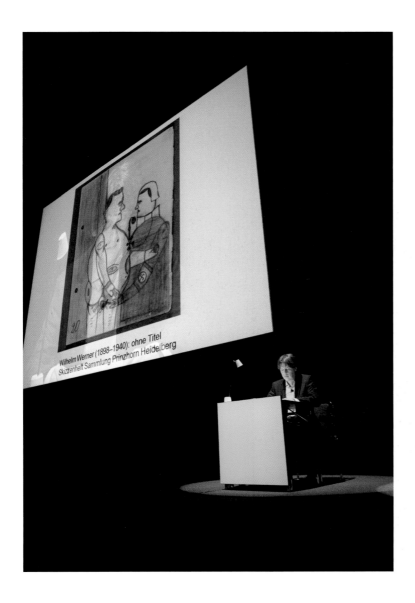

Plenary Lecture

Chair: Prof. Dr. Wolfgang Maier (Bonn), Prof. Dr. Henning Saß (Aachen)

Prof. Dr. Paul Weindling (Oxford)
Identities and Injuries – a Problematic Legacy: The Victims of Coercive Research under National Socialism in the Shadow of Psychiatry

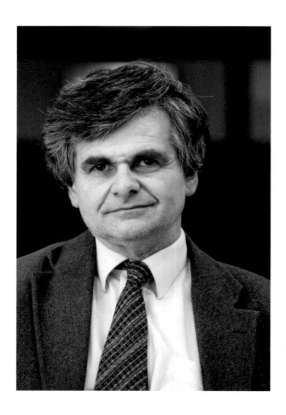

Plenarvortrag

Vorsitz: Prof. Dr. Wolfgang Maier (Bonn), Prof. Dr. Henning Saß (Aachen)

Prof. Dr. Paul Weindling (Oxford)
Identitäten und Verletzungen: Die Opfer von erzwungener Forschung im Nationalsozialismus im Schatten der Psychiatrie

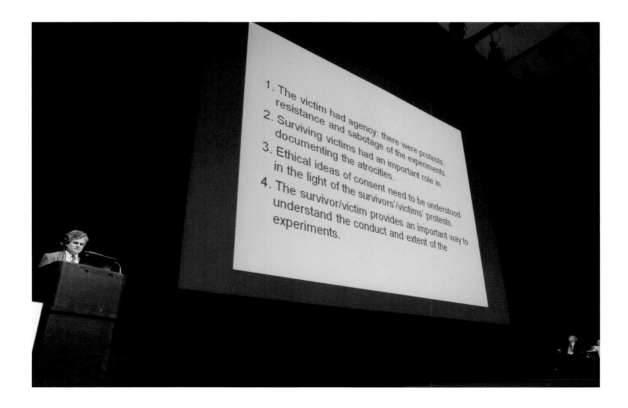

DGPPN-Scholars Congress

When doctors become perpetrators – Eugenics under the Nazi regime

What exactly went on during the period from 1933 to 1945? What does the term "eugenics" mean and what are the origins of this ideology? Can we find examples of eugenic thinking even after 1945? What are the arguments in current medical and bioethics debates? These were some of the questions that took centre stage at the DGPPN Scholars Congress on 24 November 2010 in the section focusing on the topic: When doctors become perpetrators – Eugenics under the Nazi regime.

Students prepared for the congress in advance. On the day of the Scholars Congress, Professor Michael von Cranach gave a guided tour through the "In Memoriam" exhibition as an introduction to the topic. Afterwards the students gave the presentations they had prepared for the congress, and discussed the subject in depth with Professor Volker Roelcke (Chairman of the Commission on the Investigation of the History of the DGPPN), Professor Michael von Cranach (initiator of the exhibition) and Professor Michael Seidel (head of the DGPPN's department for mental illness in patients with intellectual disabilities).

Over 100 young people attended the event in 2010. The DGPPN has been hosting student congresses as part of its annual congresses since 2003. The congresses give young people from schools in Berlin an opportunity to talk to experts about the causes, course and treatment of mental illnesses and discuss issues relating to psychiatry in their wider social context.

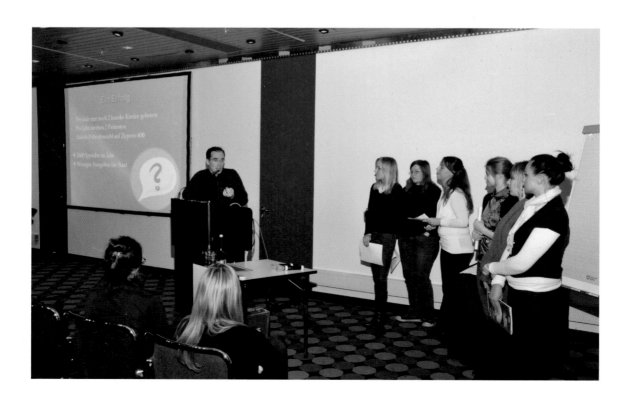

DGPPN-Schülerkongress

Wenn Ärzte zu Tätern werden: Eugenik im Nationalsozialismus

Was ist in der Zeit von 1933 bis 1945 passiert? Was bedeutet der Begriff „Eugenik" und woher kommt dieses Denken? Finden wir Beispiele eugenischen Denkens auch noch nach 1945? Welche Argumente werden in der gegenwärtigen Medizin- und Bioethik angeführt? Um diese Fragen ging es auf dem DGPPN-Schülerkongress am 24. November 2010 zum Thema „Wenn Ärzte zu Tätern werden: Eugenik im Nationalsozialismus".

Bereits im Vorfeld der Veranstaltungen beschäftigten sich die Schüler intensiv mit dem Thema. Am Tag des Schülerkongresses bot Professor Michael von Cranach den Schülern eine Führung durch die Ausstellung „In Memoriam" als Einstieg in das Thema an. Im Anschluss daran präsentierten die Schüler ihre Ergebnisse und diskutierten das Thema ausführlich mit Professor Volker Roelcke (Vorsitzender der Historischen Kommission zur Aufarbeitung der Geschichte der DGPPN), Professor Michael von Cranach (Initiator der Ausstellung) und Professor Michael Seidel (Leiter des DGPPN-Referats „Psychische Störungen bei Menschen mit geistiger Behinderung").

Insgesamt nahmen über 100 Schüler an der Veranstaltung teil. Seit 2003 bietet die DGPPN im Rahmen ihrer Jahrestagung den Schülerkongress an. Berliner Schüler erhalten die Möglichkeit, mit Experten über Ursachen, Verlauf und Therapie von psychischen Erkrankungen zu sprechen und psychiatrische Themen in ihren gesellschaftlichen Zusammenhängen zu diskutieren.

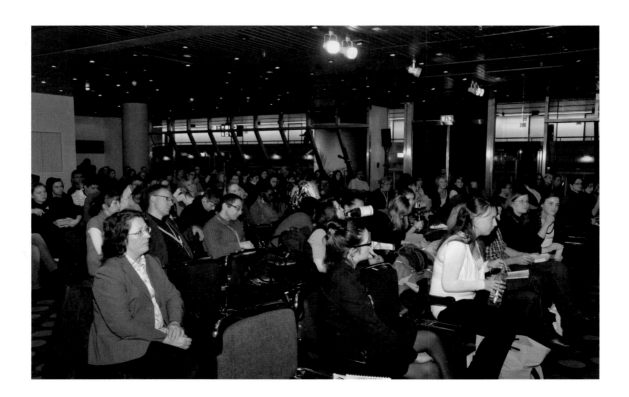

Exhibition: In Memoriam

The response among the visitors to this confrontation with the darkest chapter in the history of German psychiatry was sombre and highly contemplative.

The "In Memoriam" exhibition developed by Professor Michael von Cranach gives the victims of the Nazi's "euthanasia programmes" a face. First presented in 1999 on the occasion of the World Congress of Psychiatry in Hamburg, the exhibition was updated and expanded for the DGPPN Congress in 2010.

A dual language catalogue has been published to accompany the exhibition (von Cranach and Schneider: In Memoriam. Remembrance and responsibility, Berlin, Springer, 2010). As the preface says: "May the victims' inviolable dignity not be forgotten and may this exhibition serve to restore their own history and their own names."

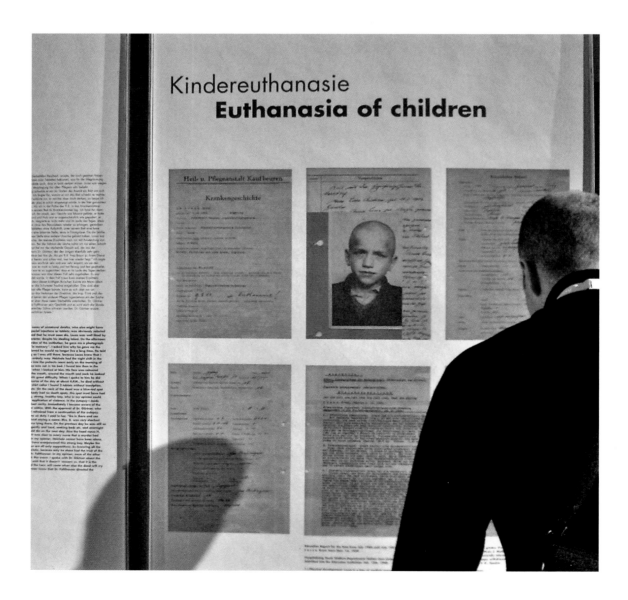

Ausstellung: In Memoriam

Die Konfrontation mit dem Schrecklichsten der Geschichte der Deutschen Psychiatrie stieß auf ein mehr als nachdenkliches Publikum.

Die von Professor Michael von Cranach entwickelte Ausstellung „In Memoriam" gibt den Opfern der nationalsozialistischen „Euthanasie-Programme" ein Gesicht. Sie wurde 1999 im Rahmen des Weltkongresses für Psychiatrie in Hamburg erstmals gezeigt und für den DGPPN Kongress 2010 erweitert und aktualisiert.

Der zweisprachige Ausstellungskatalog ist als Buch erhältlich (von Cranach und Schneider: In Memoriam. Erinnerung und Verantwortung, Berlin, Springer, 2010). Dort heißt es: „Mögen die Opfer in ihrer unantastbaren Würde nicht vergessen werden und möge die Ausstellung dazu dienen, ihnen ihre eigene Geschichte und ihren eigenen Namen zurückzugeben."

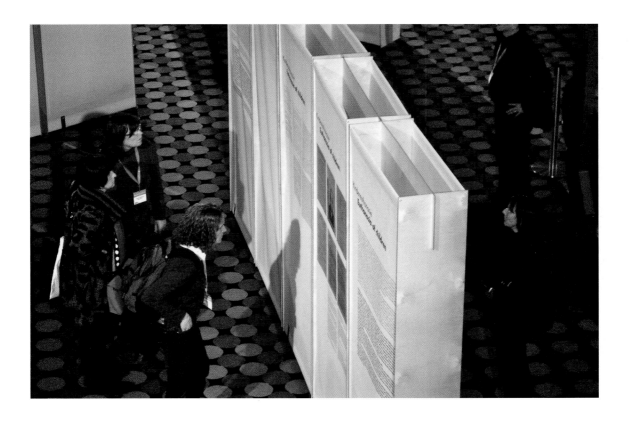

Autorenadressen / Authors addresses

Prof. Dr. med. Dr. rer. soc. Frank Schneider
Klinik für Psychiatrie, Psychotherapie und Psychosomatik
Universitätsklinikum Aachen, RWTH Aachen University
Pauwelsstraße 30
52074 Aachen
fschneider@ukaachen.de

Prof. Dr. med. Ephraim Bental
Givat Downes 33A
34349 Haifa/Israel
bental@zahav.net.il

Sigrid Falkenstein
sigrid@falkenstein-berlin.de
www.sigrid-falkenstein.de

Fotonachweis / Image credits

Ephraim Bental, Haifa: 39, 41, 47
Carsten Burfeind, Berlin: 5, 17, 22, 25, 76, 77
Sigrid Falkenstein, Berlin: 53
Andreas Kirsch, Berlin: 1/2, 18/19, 34/35, 40, 66, 74, 75
Ute Schmidt, Gelnhausen: 3, 9, 13, 23, 26, 32/33, 51, 52, 64/65, 67, 68, 69, 70, 71, 72, 73

Inhaltsverzeichnis / Table of Content

> Eine DVD mit der Videoaufnahme der Veranstaltung finden Sie am Buchende

> Please find a DVD of the commemorative event at the end of the book

Printing: Ten Brink, Meppel, The Netherlands
Binding: Stürtz, Würzburg, Germany